Physician Career Choice and Satisfaction

Empirical Studies of Practicing Physicians

Gerald D. Otis and Naomi L. Quenk

Copyright 2019 by Gerald D. Otis and Naomi L. Quenk

ISBN: 978-0-9835944-6-8

Published by Gerald D. Otis

All rights reserved. Apart from personal use by the purchaser, no part of this book may be reproduced, stored in a retrieval system, transmitted in any form or by any means (electronic, mechanical, photocopying, recording or otherwise) without prior, written consent of the copyright owner or publisher, except for the inclusion of brief quotations in an acknowledged review.

CONTENTS

	Acknowledgments	i
	Preface	iii
1	Origins and Overview	1
2	A Framework for Understanding Physician Career Choices	13
3	The Way They Were: Medical Specialties	17
4	The Way They Were: Work-settings	39
5	The Way They Were: Practice Communities	53
6	Sources of Physician Satisfaction by Specialty	63
7	Sources of Satisfaction for Practice Organizations	97
8	Psychological Type and Work-setting Characteristics	125
9	Enhancing Career Choice Using Summer Externships	135
10	Final Words	155
11	References	159
12	Appendix	167
	About the Authors	247

ACKNOWLEDGMENTS

The authors wish to express their great appreciation to John R. Graham, MD CM FRCPC DLFAPA for all his assistance and encouragement in making this volume a reality. Thanks are also due to the hundreds of medical students at the University of New Mexico and in programs managed by the American Medical Student Association Foundation as well as the hundreds of physicians in practice who took the time to fill out the many questionnaires that provided the data for most of these reports. Several others contributed, in one way or another, to the documents appearing in this book, including the now deceased Lois Dilatush, Martha Albert, and Wayne Mitchell. AMSA representatives Paul Wright and Sandy Smith provided inspiration and support during the early years. A special thanks is due Richard S. Larson, M.D., PhD., Executive Vice Chancellor and Vice Chancellor for Research at the University of New Mexico for obtaining the waiver of rights to the data collection forms described in the book.

Gerald Otis and Naomi Quenk

1 PREFACE

John R. Graham, MD CM FRCPC DLFAPA

Santa Fe, New Mexico February 2019

The thermometer was a complete surprise. Fifty years ago, I stepped out the entry door of the *new* Department of Psychiatry administrative offices at 930 Stanford Northeast. It was warm and sunny and I moved under the portal to the right side to get a better view of the extinct volcanoes and cliffs on the west mesa. When I stopped, at eye level on a supporting column, completely hidden from view of the main entry, there was an old thermometer with the same address as our office, once a marker and advertisement for the Tonnella Family Mortuary. They had death records dating back to 1932. So perhaps it was for three decades that the thermometer had dutifully measured highs and lows in temperatures and signified the building's prior life. I left it in place to continue the good work and never mentioned the thermometer to anyone. And at the end of this preface I will reveal another surprise from forty-nine years ago that I have not discussed before.

The University of New Mexico School of Medicine was the vision of President Thomas Popejoy and by 1960 he was gathering interested support from medical and political advocates for an introduction to a medical school. Initially a two-year school teaching basic sciences, with students obliged to transfer to an established four-year school out of state. I believe the first Dean of the School of Medicine and invited Department heads who had joined the faculty always were intent on the school becoming a four year independent program. There was rapid growth as basic sciences took shape and expanded. Consolidating hospital and outpatient care facilities, complete with staffing, created greater organizational upheaval when the clinical sciences were added to the educational setting.

Anticipating the 50th anniversary of the founding of the medical school, Dora L. Wang and Shannon L. Carter collected historical information, conducted interviews, and recounted events in the first phases of growth and development of the program. The resulting book *The Daily*

Practice of Compassion: A History of the University of New Mexico School of Medicine, It's People, and Its Mission, 1964 – 2014 is suggested reading on this "audacious experiment by pioneering educators who were determined to create a great medical school in a state beset by endemic poverty, and daunting geographic barriers."

Every arriving scientist and clinician wanted to create a new vision. Young professionals in the 1960's brought their dreams of a new model of medical education but, alas, their dreams rarely integrated with those of others. The unfamiliar setting led new arrivals to unwittingly, and often without conscious awareness, create a familiar face to the environment by putting versions of their prior medical school programming in place. A few seeking innovations attempted to develop the dream with varying degrees of success. Many faculty members knew the *right way*, others the *wrong way*, to accomplish the education of a medical student. Opinion based on prior experience elsewhere, rather than research findings, steered heated debate on how best to teach medicine. The student was often viewed as a container to be filled, a passive vessel to be pronounced full at some later point, rather than the vital learner entering a complicated and complex field, attempting to integrate their understanding of health and disease.

In 1961, George Miller, a dedicated physician and medical educator wrote *Teaching and Learning in Medical School*, published for the Commonwealth Fund, by Harvard University Press (ASIN:B0006AXAEW). With colleagues, foundation grants, and the support of the University of Illinois School of Medicine at the Chicago campus, the shift toward the motivation for learning emerged.

How do you learn best? How will the medical student learn best? Rather than talking about mastery of pieces of curriculum placed as obstacles on the pathway through medical education, as was the tradition, there was now consideration of the different styles of learning characterizing a variety of students; differing ideals and goals of students; an awareness that a student could have strengths and liabilities in their style of problem solving; and some dawning recognition that no single student could possibly meet all the ill-defined objectives of medical education. Changes in learning theory, applications to curriculum development, the emergence of new clinical experiences on entry to medical school, evaluation of competencies seen through the eyes and experiences of the learner, and application to the doctor-patient interactions were expressed in meaningful experiences for the student physician.

Clearly people learn best when there is a need to know more about a topic or problem. The individual as learner becomes the focus of study. And therein began the questions leading to the longitudinal study that would take place at the University of New Mexico. Planning **began in 1967. Successive cohorts of medical students who were applying to and moving through** *the black box of medical education*, **entering into postgraduate studies, and headed toward their future careers were to be tested on a variety of parameters involved with understanding and integrating a personal pathway.**

Data collection began in 1968 and captured information on the first graduates of the medical school. The support of the Division of Medical Manpower, National Institutes of Health, acquiescence of the administration of the medical school, and the enthusiasm of Gerald D Otis, PhD, Naomi L. Quenk, PhD and colleagues in the Division of Behavioral Sciences, led to a comprehensive medical education research project within the Department of Psychiatry. The tasks of longitudinal research methodology were shared with other researchers with the open invitation to work together. The Workshops at the national level, with the support of the American Association of Medical Schools and the Division of Medical Education of the American Medical Association, were held twice a year and supported for a few years by a Coordinating Office at the University of New Mexico in the 1970s.

By the mid-1980's, after the project had been terminated, there was discussion about the follow-up study to occur 20 years out from medical school graduation. With some members of the original research team, and a new project director on the full-time faculty of the school of medicine, the follow-up proposal was developed and sent off to NIH. Nothing happened. On inquiry, there was a suggestion that a reviewer at NIH did not have any interest in "researching some aging physicians." There was no understanding about longitudinal research methodology and how the follow-up measurement would allow the "secrets" to be revealed about moving through the educational continuum.

It is difficult to keep a research team alive and well over a long period of years. The drift of team members going different ways continued after the rejection of the NIH proposal. The years of effort and the absence of capstone data were sliding into oblivion.

There would never have been a follow-up of these graduates if not for the tenacity, professionalism, and expertise of Dr. Gerald Otis. On his own, without any payment or contract, Dr. Otis went through the process of collecting information about the graduates of 1968-1979 eventual career choices, connecting and collating their responses to questionnaires when they first applied to medical school. Then he set to work writing summary research results as the center focus of these reports. This concerted effort, carried across the finish line by Gerald Otis after 40-50 years becomes a remarkable statement on researcher resilience. There cannot be enough thanks provided to this dedicated research psychologist who single-handedly completed the study.

Now the present day allows an examination of the past. Gerald Otis and Naomi Quenk have combined their strengths and competencies to light up the "black box" of medical school to reveal dynamic multiple pathways through a complicated, complex, and changing set of external forces in education and patient care. There are "lights" herein for the future planning of medical education. There is a remarkable opportunity to merge research efforts at medical schools worldwide, to generate the ongoing collection and analysis of personal differences in a comprehensive database of measures with the potential of addressing global health and patient care challenges.

While anticipating the future we apply lessons from the past. Consider the context of a new school developing in the 1950s and 1960s when this longitudinal study of career pathways was taking shape. Thomas P. Duffy reviews and examines American medical education following the impact of The Flexner Report ("The Flexner Report - 100 Years Later," Yale J Biol Med, Sep: 84(3),269-276, 2011).

> "The Flexner Report of 1910 transformed the nature and process of medical education in America with a resulting elimination of proprietary schools and the

establishment of the biomedical model as the gold standard of medical training. This transformation occurred in the aftermath of the report, which embraced scientific knowledge and its advancement as the defining ethos of a modern physician.

"The Flexner Report set American medicine on a course that was fueled by the energy of scientific discovery. Those discoveries have immeasurably improved the lives of all human beings, and it is difficult to cavil in the face of such accomplishments. But the oversights of Flexner and his associates need not have occurred if these leaders had recognized the primary role of physicians as beneficent healers; the delicate balance of patient care and research could have been pursued with mutual benefits for both sides. As it was, the science of medicine eclipsed the active witnessing of our patients. Edmund Pellegrino's lament was proven true that doctors had become neutered technicians with patients in the service of science rather than science in the service of patients….

"There was maldevelopment in the structure of medical education in America in the aftermath of the Flexner Report. The profession's infatuation with the hyper-rational world of German medicine created an excellence in science that was not balanced by a comparable excellence in clinical caring. Flexner's corpus was all nerves without the life blood of caring. Osler's warning that the ideals of medicine would change as 'teacher and student chased each other down the fascinating road of research, forgetful of those wider interests to which a hospital must minister' has proven prescient and wise. We have learned that scientific medicine must travel linked to a professional ethos of caring that has been in place in our oaths and aspirations. Cross-talk must occur between the two with a bi-directional bedside to bench dialogue. This creates the frisson that animates the quest for breakthroughs in a medical realm."

The University of New Mexico was among the early leaders more than five decades ago in revisiting medical educational goals, bringing the clinical encounter between patient, and their family, in their community, into the beginning of the freshman year of medical education.

You can imagine the amount of time spent in curriculum planning in the early days of the medical school. The organ system of teaching in the basic sciences was imported to New Mexico from Case Western Reserve. With the move toward a four year accreditation, and preparation for adding on the clinical sciences, there were concerns about what was to be integrated into the first two years with basic sciences to provide relevance, and what would developing departments of clinical practice and research command in regard to the instructional time in the curriculum in the last two years of undergraduate medical education.

One multidisciplinary innovation in the clinical program was development of the Basic Clerkship in which the examination of the patient by interview, the details of the physical examination, and the approach integrating all information about medical problems were theoretically shared tasks in each of the differing medical specialties. Rather than teach something fragmented and specialized, clinical block by block, how to do a comprehensive diagnostic evaluation basic to all separate rotations through medicine, surgery, pediatrics, OB/GYN, and psychiatry was developed with all faculty acting as preceptors.

The full-scale development of the now established basic sciences, and the competing interests of the burgeoning clinical sciences combined to *start drying the concrete* of the flexible and idealized model of medical education. In 1969 a group of ten faculty members (all active and dynamic teachers) representing different basic and clinical sciences began a series of discussions planning a four year curriculum that became known as *The Cool Case and Warm Body Curriculum.*

- On entry to the medical school, the freshman student would be assigned a family in which one member had a chronic disease. The initial role of the student was to learn about the patient and their family: it was understood the medical student would be a liaison bringing family needs and medical resources together. This basic learning experience would extend over the four year educational experience inviting an understanding of the changing needs and continuing compassionate care of the individual and family within their community.

- Simultaneously the freshman student would attend an autopsy, then follow and report on all of the details of the person's death using the bridging pathological studies to lead into basic sciences and the clinical dynamics of the dying process of the patient.

- In exchange for the vibrant introduction to clinical care at the beginning of the medical school experience, a required elective in the final year would be an advanced study of basic sciences related to the individual student's developing career pathway.

Integrating the clinical encounter at the core of the New Mexico program, and bringing the basic sciences to full realization in their application to patient care was the goal of the learning experience for our graduates. And this brings me to report on a medical school faculty meeting in 1970 at the University of New Mexico. This is something I have never described before: I am keeping my promise stated at the beginning of this Preface.

My point in describing this event highlights the realities of change, particularly the *resistance* to change, as inclusive organizations attempt to remain creative, open and flexible, while institutionalization of growth can spawn *fiefdoms* struggling to hold power and control within the larger system. Individuals and like-minded persons can block central ideals and add complexities to an already complicated system. Now pardon my metaphor as I state when not dominating the larger whole, stress causes *the lords and dependent serfs* to work overtime to block progress and stimulate dry rot in the process of institutionalization. Our august curriculum committee had not anticipated what happened next.

An organized and well-written report on the *The Cool Case and Warm Body Curriculum* was prepared for the faculty to study in advance of discussion at a specially scheduled faculty meeting. By the 4 PM call to order the lecture theater was filled, more members in attendance than any previous faculty meeting in my memory.

At 4:01 the recently appointed Dean called the meeting to order and invited me to step forward to introduce the ad hoc Committee report. I was seated in the front row and before I reached the lectern, the Chair of the Department of Medicine was standing with his august colleagues and said: "I move this report be tabled."

Immediately the Chair of the Department of Surgery, amidst his white coated retinue, was standing and said, "I second the motion." With no interruption of the conversational flow, the Dean stated, "All those in favor of the motion to table say Aye," then a pause, "Those saying Nay." Then continuing, "As Chair of the Meeting I determine that the Ayes are in the majority, and the report is tabled. This meeting is adjourned."

The room was alive with talk, movement toward the exits, and confusion. The special meeting ended at 4:02 PM. There was no count of those in favor or opposed, the voice vote being interpreted by the Dean. Robert's Orders on Rules governing meetings did not set a date for the report to be taken off the table and returned to the faculty for discussion. To the best of my knowledge and during my full-time faculty appointment, there was no other Special Meeting to discuss curriculum with all faculty. The attitude of inquiry by a faculty had ended abruptly. I believe that meeting impacted the planning and development of a separate Primary Care program.

There are always changes in the needs of the population, available resources to tackle new and old problems, and technological changes that have an impact on the delivery of compassionate medical care. In the urgent push to action outcomes, combined with the seductiveness of a short-term fix in the trendiness of a medical school setting, long-term research and evidence to provide a database for decision-making is rarely considered. To the *complications* in developing responsive, responsible, and rational planning, we add the *complexities* of individual learning styles; faculty members and their committees have no time for collecting information that allows scientific *educational* research to chart excellence for graduates tracking toward multiple career pathways

When reading these reports by Otis and Quenk you cannot avoid wondering how the application of a comprehensive database tailoring a program to serve the students searching, sorting, and selecting career commitments in medicine adds vitality, self-renewal, and effectiveness to time on task. How medical education defines destinations and assists students find their pathways remains the challenge.

With the rapid technical advances bringing change in everything from individual care based on genomic medicine as an emerging medical discipline, to the impact of population growth, climate change, and the spread of treatment-resistant infections, there will always be the need for scientific information on which to plan responses to changed circumstances. Shifts in the education of new physicians, assignment of complicated tasks in new treatments, and the basic tenet that caring for the patient is the essential core of patient care have implications for education of future physicians. What a benefit longitudinal data could bring to student, educator, government, and organized medicine anticipating appropriate healthcare planning.

With the greatest respect for all the competing power centers in medicine, government, politics of every sort on the local, regional, national, and international scene I have some options for the reader and researcher to consider:

- The collective impact of medical schools working in new alliances will add efficiency to medical education and healthcare delivery in the immediate and long-term use of our limited resources

Shifting needs in our changing world will require educators and clinicians in all settings to work in a new level of trust with colleagues around this globe

- The greater good for mankind searching for peace, health, education, and living together in new relationships will stimulate new creative consortia and shared programming to improve global survival

- Longitudinal research methodology studying change over longer-term periods will be essential to responsive, reasonable, and rational interventions to maintain a careful balance between needs of the population and constraints on use of precious resources available to all countries and peoples. Should peace and cessation of violence be seen as a public health issue, imagine the advances we could make in the next fifty years for global survival, balance, meaning, and satisfaction

- Scientific data for decision making in education and life sciences will become an international necessity

The immediate application of these data drawn from longitudinal study in medical education can shape the base for development of standardized and inclusive use of techniques assisting idealistic students through the complicated and complex pathways of education to meaningful and satisfying career outcomes. Imagine the benefit to the uncertain candidate seeking counsel on career choice.

I foresee applied testing to assist students to their career goals becoming more important than National Board scores, vital markers showing progress and defining new learning tasks for our medical programs gaining cost-effectiveness in service to mankind.

With the greatest respect and thanks I commend the reader and researcher to careful reading, then application of this work by two outstanding and committed researchers with their reports as a touchstone on where we have been, and a systematic entry to discussion on where we must head immediately.

Now what are you going to do in furthering your own insights, adapting your applications of these data to provide greater good for those depending on your service and research?

Gerald Otis and Naomi Quenk

2 ORIGINS AND OVERVIEW

Gerald D. Otis

The Physician Manpower Crisis

The 1970 Carnegie Commission[1] report on medical and dental education set the stage for research on the physician workforce by declaring there was a looming health manpower deficit. Even before this report was published, Reuben A. Kessel[2], a professor of business economics at the University of Chicago, suggested that this deficit of physicians was, at least in part, an unintended consequence of the 1910 Flexner Report which had changed the standards of medical education, imposing the basic science curriculum he observed at Johns Hopkins in the first two years as the model for all medical schools. He argued that Flexner's focus on how medical students should be educated, rather than on what they should know and be able to do as a result of their education, however achieved, stifled educational innovation that would lead to more efficient ways to produce the desired output. He proposed that the basic sciences should be taught by regular academic departments before medical school and that the resources saved be used to expand enrollment of third and fourth year students. He also thought that the AMA positions antagonistic to anything but the fee-for-service model of marketing care delivery artificially restricted the availability of physicians and that their opposition to physician advertising served to maintain the high cost of medical care.

The nation responded to the claimed manpower crisis by building more medical schools, increasing enrollment, using more Advanced Placement Registered Nurses (APRNs) and more Foreign Medical Graduates (FMGs), developing new networks of care provision, and providing more funding for family practice departments and residents. Special pre-graduate programs to influence medical students to consider primary care and practice in rural and inner-city areas were instituted by the Student American Medical Association, beginning in 1968 with their Medical Education and Community Orientation (MECO) project and continuing with programs in Appalachian Health, Indian Health, Migrant Health, Health Team Training and the National Health Service Corps Primary Care Preceptorship Project. Jefferson Medical School in Pennsylvania developed a successful Physician Shortage Area Program (PSAP)[3] in 1974 that involved selective admissions, additional financial aid, a family practice advisor, a third year clerkship in family medicine in non-metropolitan areas and a senior outpatient sub-internship in family medicine.

The claim of a health manpower crisis did not go unchallenged. By 1982 the AMA, long an opponent of any governmental meddling on what they considered their turf, was asserting that "The physician shortages proclaimed by the Bane report in 1959 and the 1970 report of the Carnegie Commission on Higher Education are no longer so apparent." They believed that the "shortage" was due to an increase in demand as a result of increased average real income and the expansion of care to the poor and elderly through Medicare and Medicaid[4]. They eschewed the "forecasting and planning approach" to managing health manpower as being prone to underestimation of the ability of the health care delivery system to adjust to its changing environment. Their position was that the physician workforce was responsive to market forces, citing studies showing that communities in the 10K-20K range increased their number of physicians in five major specialties from 3 to 18%, that 18 percent of the physicians in one sample changed their medical specialty during the period between 1974-1978 and 24 percent changed their practice setting. Although acknowledging that the effects of market forces on physician manpower might be seen long after they originally occur, they believed that the decreasing financial attractiveness of medical practice and increasing educational costs to students were beginning to affect the workings of the medical education system.

A 1983 report by the Graduate Medical Education National Advisory Committee (GMENAC)[5] estimated that there would be an excess of 70,000 physicians by 1990 and recommended that U.S. Medical schools decrease enrollment by 10% relative to 1978-79 levels while also restricting the intake of FMGs. (A study of the effects of reducing enrollment in the state of Texas[6], however, concluded that it would have no significant impact on the availability of physicians over the next 15 years and might actually be counterproductive). A report by the American College of Physician Executives in 1997 stated there was increasing competition among physicians as well as hospitals for ambulatory care revenues due to the growth in enrollment of patients in integrated managed care networks. They projected a surplus of about 165,000 specialty patient care physicians by the year 2000 while they expected that the supply and demand for primary care physicians would balance out.

These predictions of a "physician glut" did not materialize in the current era. Market forces do not appear to have adequately contained the discrepancy between physician supply and demand within an acceptable time frame. In 2016 the National Center for Health Workforce Analysis, a part of the U.S. Department of Health and Human Services, using a microsimulation model with data from 2013 as a baseline, projected the supply and demand for primary care practitioners in the year 2025 for each state[7]. They expect there to be 239,460 primary care physicians in 2025 while the expected demand is 263,100 (due mainly to population growth and an aging patient group), a shortfall of 23,640 doctors. Thirty-seven states are anticipated to have a shortage of primary care physicians with 12 of them having a deficit of 1000 or more doctors. The greatest deficits are expected to be in the South (especially Florida with a need for 3,060 more than supply and Texas with a need for 1760 more than supply) while 13 states and the District of Columbia are expected to have an oversupply of primary care physicians (especially Massachusetts, with 1,230 more physicians than needed).

The Association of American Medical Colleges hired IHS Markit Ltd., a global information provider, to use a microsimulation model to infer discrepancies in physician supply and demand for the year 2030 using the 2016 level of care as a baseline[8]. Their projections were presented in terms of ranges of possibilities under different assumptions about changes in demographics, changes in insurance coverage, the amount of use of physician extenders in care delivery and changes in impediments to health care equality for under-served populations. They concluded that there would be a shortfall of between 42,600 to 121,300 physicians by 2030. Primary care physicians would fall short by between 14,800 and 49,300 while non-primary care specialists would have a deficit of from 33,800 to 72,700. Surgical specialties were expected to accrue a deficit of from 20,700 to 30,500 members due to an aging population coupled with an aging surgical workforce and a failure of surgical specialties to increase the number of new recruits. The National Council for Behavioral Health[9] in 2017 noted that the number of psychiatrists working with public sector and insured populations had declined by 10% from 2003 to 2013 due to an aging workforce, low rates of reimbursement, burnout, excessive documentation requirements and restrictive regulations about sharing clinical information. Fifty-five percent of the states have a shortage of child and adolescent psychiatrists and 77% of counties are under-served. Part of the problem with this specialty is that 40% of the psychiatric workforce provide services in cash-only private practices.

Projected numbers of physicians available and needed for different categories of physicians and places allow one to identify the *targets* for potential intervention. But additional knowledge about the physician workforce and *how its features are determined* are needed by the four entities that have a vested interest in the physician career space:

- **Medical students** need to know what options are available to them in the medical field; to know the activities and characteristics of each of these options; to know how each of them "fits" the self with regard to personal characteristics such as abilities, personality, values and interests (which also means that they need to know their own standing on these various dimensions); and to know how to make their way through the educational opportunity structure in order to attain their goals.

- **Medical schools** need to know how to select an array of different kinds of students that will, on the one hand, be capable of making it through the rigors of medical education and performing the required tasks of a physician, while, on the other hand, producing an output array of graduates who meet the array of different needs of their communities. They also need to know how to provide the kinds of teaching-learning environments that will allow different kinds of students to acquire the knowledge and skills appropriate to their different specialties and work settings. These needs presuppose that the medical school knows what kinds of graduates they want to produce in what quantities, what their communities and funding sources expect of them and that they are responsive to these expectations and not just to self-serving and guild interests.

- **Institutions and organizations that deliver health care services** need to know where to obtain the array of person-power they require in order to meet the array of demands for services in their catchment area. They also need to know the incentives that might work to attract different kinds of physicians to their facilities and the ways they might alter the activities and characteristics of their work settings to mitigate undesirable features or prepare physician-recruits to cope with them.

- ◆ **Administrative units of government** at local, state and national levels need to know how to allocate their available funds in order to help different kinds of medical care providers to meet the needs of their constituents in various locals, especially those characterized by low income and rural location. They need to know what contingencies they may most appropriately require for allocating funds to communities or health care facilities, what kinds of incentives they may make available in order to attract the needed kinds of physicians to their state or region, and how to craft legislation that will actually help them to achieve their health care goals.

Of course these different entities also need other kinds of information to make their decisions (e. g., amount of demand for different kinds of services, impending alterations in organization of health care delivery, changes in disease frequencies and new treatment options that may be in the offing, degree to which paramedical personnel may be substituted for physicians, etc.). But they all need to know how to find different kinds of students or physicians, how to select them, and how to influence or coax them into the kinds of activities and settings where they are needed.

Enter The Longitudinal Study

The Longitudinal Study emerged just as debate about how to solve the manpower problem was getting heated. The University of New Mexico School of Medicine was in its infancy when I joined the Behavioral Sciences Training Group in the Department of Psychiatry in 1966. Graduation of the medical school's first crop of physicians was still two years away and during that time, many new faculty and facilities were added. We went from being housed in a converted mobile home to offices in the newly formed Psychiatry building, which earlier had been the medical school mortuary.

One of the new psychiatrists, John R. Graham, MD who had a long-standing interest in developing a fact-based and rational approach to medical education, called a meeting of those who might have an interest in developing a research project to study physicians in training and the process of medical education. The late Lois Dilatush, our sociologist, and I showed up. Dr. Graham mentioned a couple of studies by L. Eron that had found an increasing amount of "cynicism" as students went through medical school, a situation that might have adverse effects on the way they practiced medicine and the outcomes of their encounters with patients. That sounded important to all of us present, so we decided to initiate a longitudinal study of medical students as they developed into physicians. Our initial focus was on attitudes toward psychosocial aspects of medicine and any changes in those attitudes, if they could be established empirically.

At the same time, the national concern about the "maldistribution of physician manpower" was occurring. It was asserted, by both politicians and leaders of the medical community, that there were too few primary care physicians, that too few practiced in small communities and the inner city, and that certain kinds of work-settings had chronic problems in recruiting sufficient physician manpower. Somehow, individuals at the Bureau of Health Manpower learned that we were collecting career preference information and paid us a visit, leading to a series of federal contracts, beginning in 1970.

Although we had been interested in medical career development in general, the advent of federal funding focused our efforts on the selection of medical specialty, practice setting, and nature of the community in which to practice. These areas had become salient, at the time, as government officials, educators and program planners struggled with the problem of how to match the nation's output of physician manpower with the heterogeneous "map" of the needs for their services.

In the next few years, we assembled a very talented, enthusiastic and creative team consisting of two psychologists, a sociologist, three graduate students in education, several research assistants, a nurse researcher, clerical staff, and computer programmers. Over the years, a method of working together emerged that was similar to a matrix management system: the nature of the tasks to be performed and the knowledge, skills, and talents of the individuals involved determined who had authority and responsibility for particular activities. The "director" for one project might be the assistant for another project. Because certain kinds of tasks were recurring and certain individuals had strengths in different areas, there was superimposed on the matrix system a more constant division of labor for some activities. We ended up being located in a house purchased by the University about a block from the main medical school campus. That allowed us to take coffee breaks, tend the roses, or play badminton in the back yard. And the research team often celebrated holidays together with feasts in which everyone would contribute some part of the meal. Years after the project was terminated, former team members said that, except for the pay, it was the best job they had ever had.

Looking back on it, it is interesting to note the rapid changes that took place technologically. We went from keeping student data on handwritten spreadsheets and analyzing them using a programmable Wang calculator, to key-punching data on computer cards and carting large boxes of such cards over, first to the Kirkland Air Force Base CDC 6600 computer and later to the smoke-filled UNM Computer Center with its IBM 360. There, an interpreter machine would read the cards, often chewing them up or throwing out cards it didn't like. Eventually we moved to tape and finally disk storage (although the disks at that time were about 14 inches in diameter).

Over its nine years of operation, the Longitudinal Study developed several sources of data. The first, of course, was that collected from medical students just prior to entry into medical school and then repeated at the end of each year of medical school and, eventually, beyond medical school to graduate medical training and practice itself. These data included: information on personality characteristics and preferences; current status of preferences for a wide range of medical specialties and practice situations; student's expectations and perceptions of student-faculty relationships; students notions of desirable and undesirable physician characteristics; background and demographic characteristics potentially relevant to career aspirations; and, after graduation, information about internships, residencies, medical practice experiences and preferences. (Descriptions of all of the data collection instruments, as well as the instruments themselves, are presented in the appendix.)

The Study also collected data from faculty on their expectations and perceptions of student-faculty relations, using an appropriately modified version of the instrument used to assess students. In addition, data was collected on a large national sample of physicians in practice in order to develop a taxonomy of physician work settings. A separate sample of personality characteristics of teachers and residents in family practice was collected. And a database of publicly available information on all US medical schools was obtained in order to establish a typology of medical schools and relate it to the schools' output of different types of physicians.

Finally, we developed a long collaborative relationship with the American Medical Student Association (AMSA) Foundation. We obtained and analyzed data on medical students placed in summer medical externships to assess the influence of their experiences on areas related to career and work-setting choice and fed back the results to program coordinators so they could fine-tune their placements to optimize certain effects.

There are many classes of "entities" involved in the physician "career space": medical students, medical schools, departments within medical schools, medical specialties, physician work settings, practice communities, incentive programs and programs meant to influence medical students in one way or another. There probably are others that we did not investigate. The entities within these classes vary, one to another, in terms of their values on the properties (attributes, characteristics, parameters) associated with the entities and these values may co-vary with one another, bound together on the basis of some underlying set of dimensions of variation. One objective, then, was to map out the dimensions of variation in property values for the various entities. Another objective was to identify any unusual concentrations of individuals in the multidimensional score spaces ("kinds" or "types" of entities). The third objective was to assess any linear relationships between these dimensions and our dependent variables of interest and non-linear relationships between types and dependent variables of interest (usually, but not always, choice of specialty, work-setting or community in which to practice). Our "hypotheses" regarding casual agents or influences were manifested in what we chose to measure, based on theory, previous research, past experience or intuition.

Many interim articles, monographs, and reports resulted from the analyses of these various data sets. However, in 1976, the government, in its infinite wisdom, decided to "solve" the problem of physician maldistribution by fiat: they just declared that there wasn't a problem because the majority of individuals in the population lived within 50 miles of a physician and other specialists could do what generalists could do. Actually, it seemed, they had just become weary of dealing with the problem and wanted to devote their resources to something else. Nevertheless, some members of the medical community and sometimes even government planners would raise the issue about every five years thereafter, it appearing and soon fading from view in newspaper accounts when no one would take up the challenge. It is still in the news in substantially the same form in 2019 as it was in the 1970s.

For the medical student data, the termination of the project left several limitations due to the fact that many graduates were still "in process" and not actually engaged in medical practice. Thus, we could not determine what specialties, work settings, or communities they eventually chose since they had not yet made those choices. Other limitations were imposed by the time period that certain assessment instruments were introduced into the project, i. e., some subjects had already passed through some stages of education before we started using the instrument. Thus, it was not possible, soon after the end of the project, to engage in many fruitful analyses.

An appeal for funds ($2000) from the medical school to keep the data collection going was denied, so the project director and the senior staff decided to take up the AMSA Foundation's offer to set us up as an independent Center for Physician Career Development. However, after a couple of years, the AMSA Foundation also succumbed to the same government shortsightedness and financial problems as did the Longitudinal Study. After that, the researchers' professional careers took different paths and the Longitudinal Study was forgotten.

But the student data was retained and lived on in each of my personal computers for the next few decades. I occasionally would run some analyses on it and in the early years of the Internet would try to locate some of our graduates, but at that time it was hit and miss. A couple of times, the "father" of the study, John R. Graham, MD, and I tried to stimulate the medical school to help in a follow-up study but these efforts went nowhere. It was not until I had retired and been recruited to help Dr. Graham with research on his grade school mentoring program, MATCH New Mexico, that I was again inspired to "do something" with the Longitudinal Study data.

I started by seeing how many graduates I could find on the Internet, which had improved vastly since the early days. I surprised myself when I was able to locate 86% of matriculating students during the Longitudinal Study era. I noted their specialties and then went back to see if I could figure out their practice type and was able to cast them into one of eight categories most of the time. For population size, I obtained the population on Wikipedia for their designated place of practice and then checked on a map to make sure it was not a suburb of a large metropolitan area. If so, it was classified with the largest of the four population categories. Then I began to analyze the specialty, work-setting and community size categories with respect to the data collected during the original Longitudinal Study. The results detailed the relationships between information obtained at the time of acceptance to medical school (but before starting classes) and the physicians' specialties, work-settings and communities some 50 years later.

I reviewed some of our earlier work and began to think it should not just disappear, since much of it was never published and it appeared to still be relevant to current problems in managing physician manpower and providing guidance for new studies of the physician production system. The Longitudinal Study had offered three frameworks for considering the differentiation of medical students as they traverse the medical education territory.

- ◆ The first was a general framework in which medical student efforts and activities during medical school were seen in the context of *concept formation and problem solving*. That is, during medical school, students learn and modify concepts at various levels of abstraction, whether they be represented mentally as enactments, icons or verbal/symbolic forms, whether they be the concepts of common sense or scientific ones, whether they be about the self, the ideal self, the feared self or objects outside the self. And they use these concepts to solve the problems presented to them in life, including the problems of selecting a specialty, work setting or community in which to practice.

- The second formulation considered the medical student as an *object of professional socialization*, a person seeking an optimum match between the career alternatives open to him/her and his/her own preferences and life circumstances. The elements conceptualized in this process were the personal characteristics domain, the cognitive lens, the medical school environment, and the choice domain.
- The third formulation considered medical students as being sorted into different subpopulations as they pass through *an opportunity structure* that involves making choices at various stages and having some of their attributes transformed as a result of being exposed to different environments from the ones they didn't choose. Eventually, after an extensive series of sortings, the medical student ends up in a particular specialty, a particular work-setting and a particular community.

Pre-choice affinities (and aversions) to particular specialties, work-settings and communities were conceptualized as *dispositions* varying in magnitude and valence and measurable on seven-point approach–avoidance scales. Intercorrelations of these dispositions revealed which ones "went together" and factor analysis sorted these into different relatively independent dimensions or "variable clusters." Like-minded groups of students were identified by finding patterns of scores across these several dimensions and these *patterns of approach-avoidance* were found to predict ultimate career choice more precisely than did relying on simple first choice preferences. The patterns were also found to be significantly related to outside variables, i. e., those not used to define them, such as attitudes and personality characteristics.

A similar approach of identifying dimensions of co-variation and subgroups of cases with similar patterns of scores on the resulting dimensions was used to identify types of medical students, types of medical schools, types of physician work-settings, and "experiential" types of students who participated in MECO preceptorship programs. The many ways in which the types so-identified differed from the group as a whole were determined through Monte-Carlo analyses in which the means of each group were compared to the means of numerous random samples of liked-sized groups taken from the total population of scores on a set of external variables. Thus:

- Twelve types of medical students were identified on the basis of personality characteristics and were found to "stand out" from the total group with respect to academic ability and performance, preferred methods of learning, perceived goals of the medical school, expectations and perceptions of student-faculty relations, physician ideology, career preferences and use of leisure time.
- Six of the ten types of medical schools identified by scores on five dimensions of institutional characteristics were found to have different rates of production of medical specialties, medical school faculty and researchers.
- Patterns of scores on seven dimensions of physician work-setting characteristics from 413 practicing physicians produced seven physician "niches" and were related to differential rates of satisfaction and to aspects of their practice they would like to see be more or less characteristic.
- Score patterns on six program dimensions based on student ratings of the amount of exposure

they had to different program activities in their MECO preceptorship program resulted in ten "experience types" and each of these types were significantly different from the total group in their initial specialty and career interests, subsequent career inclinations, medical attitudes, goal achievements, and ratings of the degree of negativity, disillusionment and helpfulness they had of their MECO programs.

Numerous other analyses were performed to address specific topics of interest in the physician workforce arena.

- ◆ Medical school faculty from different departments were found to present different "images" to medical students in terms of their physician ideology and the way they perceive and interact with students. It is suspected that the images projected by faculty members become associated with the specialties they represent and, for the student, aid in differentiating his or her own professional identity. It might be argued, therefore, that personality, value, attitudinal and stylistic differences in specialists are functional aspects of the medical school environment and are necessary for the professional development of the student.

- ◆ Over the course of medical school, students appear to weed out specialty options from a "neutral" category and place them into "negative" and sometimes positive categories. The largest effect occurs in years 3 and 4 as students get direct exposure to different specialty milieus during their clerkship rotations. Direct experience with the tasks of different specialties, as occurs in clinical clerkship rotations, appears to be important in evaluating the "fit" of the various specialties but may occur after the date that the student has to commit to a particular residency program. It might be possible for such experiences to be presented in abbreviated form or via some sort of simulation earlier in the course of medical education.

- ◆ An exercise in numerical model building created a first stage model of physician career dispositions that linked together 36 variables representing student characteristics on entry to medical school, 11 variables representing student experiences during medical school, and 40 variables representing senior medical student career dispositions. Operation of the model was illustrated by making hypothetical changes in the values of one or more student input and experiential variables and observing the effects produced on the array of senior career dispositions. Outcomes of these simulation runs was consistent with what was known from the literature or suspected by experience to result from such changes. However, it was concluded that the further development of such models require more conceptual development.

    A model necessarily represents a process of abstraction but that process is not so simple when one is attempting to model a group of sensate beings, all of whom are different, all of whom selectively process, store, cumulate and review information from their experience and an environment that is quite non-homogeneous when described in the terms of everyday language. Add on to this the condition that one is interested in many output variables and the situation becomes almost overwhelming. It is like asking the aircraft engineer to model a formation of aircraft flying in mountainous terrain during a thunderstorm, each plane headed for different destinations and taking into account not only aerodynamic performance characteristics but also a multitude of stress tolerance factors, passenger comfort, and so on.

> What is needed to handle this complexity is the development of a set of middle and higher level concepts that transcend idiosyncrasies of individual experience and the uniqueness of medical schools or other institutions and concepts that allow one to factor the problem into a set of simpler problems. While concepts at these levels of abstraction are beginning to be developed in parts of sociology and political science, there is not even a beginning in the field of physician career development. Time and energy devoted to such an effort would seem to be a wise investment.

As a result of this review, I decided to create a collection of papers containing most of the several studies we had carried out previously as well as the new follow-up study. The result was an unwieldy document with 28 chapters, numerous hyper-links and spanning some 650 pages. But then obstacles to publication began to appear.

When permission was sought for reprinting some of the studies that had been published years before in journals, it was discovered that either I was not allowed to do so (even with my own publications) or it was prohibitively expensive. Academic publishing had changed considerably since I last was involved; journals had sold off rights to publishers who offered the articles as pay-per-view items on the Internet and they wanted no competition from the authors of those articles nor did they feel obligated to pay royalties to them. I learned that only a particular "presentation" of results of scientific investigations could be copyrighted, not the results themselves. So I either used earlier versions of the papers or rewrote them as different "presentations" in order to get around that obstacle. Since I had wanted to include the various instruments we had created to gather data (even though they were never copyrighted), I had to obtain a waiver from the university for their inclusion, which took two months to accomplish because the person who was supposed to handle my initial request had left the institution.

I had wanted to publish the book as an open access document in order to reduce or eliminate financial impediments to its distribution but, when I started looking at the fine print, I learned that these publishers were not really free either. They charge authors an "article processing charge" (APC) up front which they assume can be recovered by the author from his funding source or the institution with which he is affiliated. Since I am retired, I have no funding source and I no longer have an affiliation with an institution. I would also have had to sign up with ORCID, a organization that provides a digital identifier for researchers, something I neither need nor want. Nor did I need "peer review" of my research. If you can't understand the material and think for yourself, do not read any further. I just wanted to skip all the nonsense and make the information available to the public.

Having already published several books on Amazon and Barnes & Noble, I was acquainted with the procedures involved in self publishing, so I opted for that venue, limiting the content of the book to manageable (and printable) proportions by focusing on student characteristics associated with subsequent career choices, characteristics and satisfactions associated with different specialties and work settings, and efforts designed to influence the career decision process.

An Overview

While the Longitudinal Study was born out of a concern about the apparent development of increasingly cynical attitudes of medical students during the period of their education, the Zeitgeist together with financial support provided by the federal government soon focused the project on the mechanisms of production of different kinds of physicians, identifying the various forces that contribute to graduates choosing a set of options from amongst their career alternatives. We assumed there was a numerical deficit in physician production relative to demand for their services and that there were maldistributions of physicians in certain specialties, work settings and communities along the lines of those that were specified. But we allowed as to how the particular deficits of the day might change in the future due to the complex dynamics of the medical care system and thus, looking ahead to the long-term information needs, we thought we should consider the whole array of specialties, work settings and communities rather than just those that currently show a deficit. This has proven to be at least partially true as there are, many years later, an apparent deficit in psychiatrists and (probably) surgeons as well as the continuing deficit in practitioners of primary care and those practicing in small communities.

- ◆ The first chapter after this one provides an abbreviated version of Mitchell's model of physician career choice as an orienting framework for the studies that follow.

- ◆ Three chapters present the results of the half-a-century-later follow-up study of Longitudinal Study medical students. What did our graduates eventually decide in terms of specialty, work-setting and community choices? Using data collected upon entry to medical school, 86% of the participants in the original study were traced on the Internet and their specialty, work-setting and community size were determined. Mean values on a large number of the measures collected upon entry to medical school "stood out" (i. e., were statistically significant) for each of the seven specialty groups, eight practice organization groups, and four population size groups. These measures included personality test scores, measures of physician ideology, student-faculty role expectations, measures of academic ability and performance, career dispositions and background information.

    Students who ended up practicing in different specialties, work settings and size communities were shown to have measurably different characteristics at the beginning of medical school and to perform differently in medical school and on National Boards Examinations. Medical students who eventually chose a specialty within the Family Medicine Cluster were the only group of students to anticipate their eventual specialty with a high degree of accuracy from the time they were admitted to medical school on through to graduation. In the work-setting domain, only students who eventually ended up practicing in institutions (hospitals, universities and government facilities) were able to accurately anticipate their work setting at the time they entered medical school. Fifty-six percent of the small town practitioners were predictable from their entry level ratings of 15 practice community characteristics while 86% of those practicing in a large city knew that would be their destination from the start.

- ◆ In a national sample of 477 physicians in practice, regression analysis was used to compute the percent of variance in satisfaction that could be accounted for in 13 different specialties on the basis of practice characteristics, personality and demographic features. While the percent of variance accounted for in physician satisfaction across all specialties was only 16%, the average for the individual specialties was an impressive 65%, with Ob-Gyn and surgery being the most predictable while pediatrics was least predictable.

◆ Many significant differences were found when satisfied physicians were compared with dissatisfied physicians in eight different practice organizations. While the variance accounted for in most of the practice organizations averaged about 50% or less, nearly all of it was predictable in non-governmental hospitals. Full-time V.A. physicians were found to be more dissatisfied with their total situation than their part-time colleagues. The characteristics of full-time V.A. employment appear to be inherently dissatisfying to many physicians. Several factors are at play including control, administrative structure, a large underbelly of decision-making fiefdoms, and a lot of "difficult" patients with substance abuse and emotional disorders.

◆ Many characteristic and activities in physician work-settings are significantly related to Psychological Type as measured by the Myers-Briggs Type Indicator (MBTI), e. g. some types have greater incomes and engage in larger amounts of direct patient care than do other types. Family practice teachers and residents are different from the general medical population in terms of MBTI Type but a greater percentage of the residents are Sensing-Judging types while their teachers are more heavily represented by Intuitive-Feeling types. It is also interesting to note that different Psychological Types of medical students performed better or worse on different sub-tasks in an evaluation of a course in clinical problem solving.

◆ As examples of programs designed to influence career dispositions of medical students, Medical Education and Community Orientation (MECO) programs that were organized by the American Medical Student Association Foundation were generally perceived by participants as successful in helping them learn about career options, attracting them to the communities in which they had their preceptorship experiences, increasing their knowledge about the medical care system and clinical-technical aspects of medicine. The experiences bring about certain kinds of changes in career dispositions, especially those connected with work settings and tend to occur for all MECO participants during their projects. The amount of change in certain kinds of specialty and practice community dispositions as well as the amount of perceived success for different goals was dependent upon both student characteristics and program characteristics. Using path analysis, the size of community of origin, size of preceptorship community, and initial dispositions toward practicing in small communities were found to significantly affect post-preceptorship dispositions toward small town practice. The major portion of the effect of size of community of origin appeared to be indirect, due to its effect on the other variables.

From this preview, it can be seen that there are many pathways connecting various points of interest in the map of physician career space. The Longitudinal Study has touched on some of them but many are yet to be discovered and elaborated upon.

It is hoped that these short descriptions of the results of the research will whet the appetite of the reader for more in-depth discovery by reading the full chapters from which they are drawn.

2 A FRAMEWORK FOR UNDERSTANDING PHYSICIAN CAREER CHOICES

Gerald D. Otis

The late Wayne Mitchell, PhD joined the Longitudinal Study team a few years after it had started. A sociologist with a strong statistical background and a bent toward combining both sociological and psychological perspectives, he worked on most areas of the project but especially our mathematical modeling effort. Mitchell's contributions were many, including a reconceptualization of Restle's mathematical choice model, and development of an approach to creating ratio scales for assessment of physician career dispositions. The Longitudinal Study, in its early years, was largely an empirical endeavor because there was no theory of the process of physician career decision making to provide guidance. Of course, we had our hunches about what was relevant and these were implicit in our selection of instruments and development of scales. What Mitchell did was to make our implicit assumptions explicit and to create a formulation of the process that would help guide our research efforts [10].

One general assumption was that degree of satisfaction with a career choice depended on the degree of correspondence between a person's preferences and priorities, on the one hand, and the features of a career niche that afforded realization of those preferences and priorities, on the other. These properties or qualities of an object or environment that define its possible uses have been called "affordances." For example, a chair affords the possibility of sitting down on it. A medical student would thus try to select a career niche that possessed features that he believed would optimize this correspondence between work environment and self (and therefore his overall satisfaction). This would, of course, occur within the limitations imposed by the student's abilities and life circumstances. In order to make this attempt, the student would need to know information about himself, information about the affordances of career niches, and have a mechanism to calculate the degree to which the alternative niches would foster realization of his self. A further assumption was that the medical student acquires this information, about both self and niche, through his medical training experiences.

Mitchell proposed that the components involved in this matching process include the personal characteristics domain, the cognitive lens, the educational environment, and the choice domain.

Within the personal characteristics domain are *past experiences* that help configure personality, world view, values and interests; *present life circumstances* that include a number of status variable such as marital status, financial status, age, religion, occupation of spouse, number of children; *personality* or those relatively stable psychological characteristics that determine style and adaptation; and *attitudes, beliefs, values and predispositions,* i. e., more immediate precursors of action or behavior which are presumably more malleable than personality traits.

The cognitive lens determines what parts of his environment or what sorts of information the individual focuses on and how he or she will search for information. It is a function of both personality and experience.

The range of information and experiences the student is exposed to is determined by the educational environment and it is composed of two aspects: the *mirror* and the *prism*. The mirror reflects back to the student an image of himself, his strengths and weaknesses, as a result of judgments made about him by faculty. It also allows him to compare himself to other students and faculty and make his own judgments about his strengths and weaknesses. The nature of the specialties, types of practice, values and attitudes are refracted through the prism and colored by the beliefs, attitudes and values of other students and faulty.

The choice domain is composed of career niches which include sub-components of specialties, work settings, type of community and distribution of work effort. Prior to actual experience in such environments, the student can only know about them through the images he gets of them as provided by his training experience. The matching process is a dynamic one because components of his personal characteristics change, i. e., his abilities, values, confidence, knowledge base. And his perceptions and understandings (and sometimes the reality) of niche characteristics also change. One implication of all this variability is that prediction of career dispositions from characteristics assessed early in the process may not be as strong as from those assessed later and there may be dramatic fluctuations over time. The model would suggest that upsurges and down-turns in student interest in certain areas of medicine are likely due to exposure to new experiences (as in clerkships) or to particularly influential faculty role models who may give students a memorable but distorted image of a given area of medical practice.

This highest level of conceptualization is very abstract, as Mitchell noted, and tells us where to look and what to look at but does not have the kind of specification and detail to generate testable hypotheses. The next lower level of abstraction, Level II, is that of *mid-range theories* that specify constructs, assumptions and propositions. "Constructs" are concepts that are created by researchers so as to restrict the scope of the investigation and permit delineation of more specific assumptions, testable hypotheses and empirical inquiry. This is the level at which theories are verified or disconfirmed and constructs and propositions are modified as the result of findings at Level III.

Level III is the level where the constructs and propositions of Level II get operationalized, i. e., get cast into a form where measurements of the constructs and propositions can be made, even if it is just nominal (presence/absence) measurement. Thus, a construct such as Introversion might get represented by scores on a personality inventory or a disposition toward a specialty might get represented by a rating on a seven point scale of attraction/repulsion from that specialty. This is the level where the degree of conformity to reality of the theoretical propositions is tested, usually with some kind of statistical procedure. If the results of these tests indicate that the theoretical propositions of Level II are too discrepant from reality, they might be revised or a different set of constructs might be employed to implement the categories of Level I. Then the testing procedure is carried out again and repeated until confirmatory results are obtained. That is, the empirical data at Level III provides feedback that the researcher can use to improve and possibly expand his theoretical developments at level II, the middle range. Tinkering with the assumptions, constructs and propositions of the middle range is how construction of a viable theory takes place. Mitchell refers to Level I as a model but I prefer to call it a "framework" since the term "model" is also used to refer to mathematically specified relationships between constructs like in path diagrams or econometric models of some phenomena. The function of the framework is to point to content areas (e. g., personality, career dispositions, constraints, choice theories, and socialization theories) of middle range theories or propositions that can be linked together so as to increase our understanding of the niche selection process.

Mitchell illustrates the process of theory building by incorporating Jung's theory of psychological types and a choice theory into the framework. Jung's type theory proposes that there are different kinds of people in the world based upon certain bipolar distinctions in their mental functions and orientations to the world. In the realm of perception, he proposed two approaches: perceiving (P) and sensing (S). In the realm of judgment, he proposed two varieties: thinking (T) and feeling (F). With regard to global orientations to the world, he proposed those who were introverted (I) or extraverted (E). Isabel Myers added a fourth contrast between judging (J) and perceiving (P) based on a person's attitude toward the *outside* world of people and things. Concatenation of these contrasts yield a matrix of 16 types of people who differ in their operating characteristics, phrased in terms of their preferences and dispreferences for different types of activities and their usual acquisition of certain kinds of skills and talents. Thus, ESTJs like to organize and systematize things, prefer working with things that are physically "real" and unambiguous, like decisive action, and tend to become good managers of operations. Translating these general kinds of preferences into the medical career realm, one would expect these kinds of medical students to prefer specialties like surgery or technique and instrument oriented specialties (e. g., ophthalmology) rather than psychiatry or neurology. Their psychological opposites, the INFPs, are psychologically-minded, prefer complex problem solving, and want to help others realize their potential. They would be expected to be drawn to psychiatry and some aspects of family practice. Other predictions in the medical career preference realm could be made for many other types, thereby expanding the nomological network of the theory, i. e., the representation of the concepts, their observable manifestations, and the interrelationships among and between them.

The assumption, at Level I, that students will change in their preferences as they gain more knowledge about themselves and the career niches in the field of medicine, when combined with the knowledge of differential operating characteristics of the different psychological types, leads to even greater elaboration of the Level II theory. The ESTJs, for example, might be expected to arrive at more stable career preferences earlier in their education because they tend to make judgments – arrive at decisions – sooner than other types. On the other hand, the INFPs tend to delay decision-making so as to be sure they have touched base with all the possibilities. This hypothesis of differential decision times might also apply to other aspects of career decision making such as allocation of professional effort into different tasks (clinical care, research, administration), choice of practice community and choice of work setting.

More complicated propositions are also suggested by the specification of this particular personality theory in the theory of physician career choice. For example, introverted thinking types (IT's) are less disposed toward informal socialization with faculty and therefore may have less exposure to sources of detailed information about certain specialties and work-settings than the more gregarious extraverted feeling types (EF's).

Mitchell made the distinction between qualitative and quantitative choice theories. Qualitative theories consider choices to be made on the basis of what features are present or absent in the alternatives while quantitative theories view choice as dependent on the degree to which the features are thought to be present. Qualitative theories may work best when the alternatives are highly unalike or the chooser has a limited amount of information about the alternatives. Quantitative theories, on the other hand, may function best when the individual has a lot of information about the alternatives and he or she has limited the number of alternatives being considered. Applying this distinction to our medical student career choosers, we might expect them to rely on qualitative paradigms early in their education when they have little information about the characteristics of the alternatives while, later in their education when they have acquired more information about the features associated with the alternatives, they may rely more on quantitative models to express their preferences.

If both personality and choice theories are both incorporated into the mid-range theory of niche selection in medicine we might consider how different personality types differ in their preferences for simplicity (taking account of only a few attributes associated with each alternative) as opposed to complexity (using combinations of several characteristics) in decision-making. Given that processing combinations of attributes is likely to take longer than processing just a few, one might expect introverted perceiving types, who like to reflect at length before deciding, to arrive at their stable career choice later than other types. The point here is that, if we know the kinds of decision models different types prefer, we can expand the theory to include phenomena that might otherwise not be considered.

Mitchell believed that his conceptualization of the process of medical career choice provided a cohesive framework within which a variety of results could be unified. It is flexible and open enough that it does not exclude potentially fruitful areas of study yet it also provides enough of a structure that it can, to some degree, direct research efforts. It also allows researchers to select or create different constructs and propositions within the categories of Level I, try them out and test them to evaluate which are the most useful.

3 THE WAY THEY WERE: MEDICAL SPECIALTIES

Gerald D. Otis

Choice of medical specialty has been a subject of empirical inquiry for decades and continues to be of interest to researchers, developers of medical school curricula and health care planners[11, 12]. Bowman[13] has looked at the relationship between career choice and health policy initiatives over the last four decades and found that, in spite of a substantial increase in numbers of primary care physicians, there has been a decrease in "standard primary care years per graduate" in both physicians and physician extenders. The "institutional types" of medical schools that produce physicians[14] as well as various exposure[15] programs for primary care have been studied. Personality factors have been extensively studied and have produced a number of characteristics somewhat inconsistently associated with different medical specialties[16, 17].

Medical students can be considered as possessing "nascent images" of their future medical careers, with some features of the image tentatively decided, some still unspecified, and all of them subject to modification with the advent of new experience. The degree to which medical students' nascent images are able to anticipate their eventual specialty choice has become a topic of debate because of proposals to shorten the length of medical education by developing tracks for students headed in different directions.[18, 19, 20, 21, 22, 23]

This study was a 50 year follow-up of the UNM Medical School graduates described in earlier chapters. The initial list of medical students totaled 542 individuals of whom 465 were located on the Internet who had specialty, work-setting and community information available. They were traced using Bing and Google searches which usually resulted in several "hits" to a professional web site, a repository of physician information (Healthgrades, Vitals, Doximity, etc.) or some other location (e. g., medical school). Their identities were confirmed by locating the date of graduation from UNM listed on the web site. If the identity could not be confirmed, the case was dropped from the sample. From one or more web sites, the physician's specialty was determined as well as her/his work-setting and location of practice. Half of the students remained to practice in the Rocky Mountain Region with an additional 22% moving to the West Coast and 11% practicing in the West South Central Region (mostly Texas). Thirty one percent of found graduates ended up practicing in New Mexico and 59% of those practiced in Albuquerque.

Methods

Participants self-identified into one of 18 specialties: Otolaryngology (1%), Orthopedics (3%), Internal Medicine (15%), Pathology (6%), Obstetrics-gynecology (6%), Pediatrics (7%), Cardiology (2%), Psychiatry (7%), Allergy (1%), Family Medicine/General Practice (20%), Ophthalmology (3%), Preventive Medicine (2%), Surgery (7%), Dermatology (4%), Radiology (4%), Emergency Medicine (7%), Anesthesiology (4%) and Neurology (5%). Compared to the percentages from the *AAMC 2012 Physician Specialty Data Book*[14], the only figures that stand out are for Internal Medicine (3.5% higher than the national group) and Family Medicine (7.7% higher than the national group).

In order to reduce the number of specialty categories and therefore increase the number of cases within categories, specialties were combined into clusters of "similar" specialties. The categories of specialties and sub-specialties formally claimed by internal medicine and surgery professional associations did not appear to be psychologically meaningful. Instead, specialties were grouped on the basis of a factor analysis of ratings of specialty inclination made by these students in their final year of medical school. One cluster was dropped because it was an empty class when cases with missing data were excluded. (It should be noted that the factor analysis was just used to establish what specialties belonged together; the objects being classified were the practicing physicians). The seven categories that ended up being used were:

1. Cluster 1 IM: general internal medicine, pulmonology, cardiology and gastroenterology (n = 80, 17%).

2. Cluster 2 SURG: general surgery, orthopedic surgery, plastic surgery, thoracic surgery, urology, neurosurgery (n = 49, 11%).

3. Cluster 3 FM: family practice, pediatrics, general practice, emergency medicine, public health (n = 153, 33%).

4. Cluster 4 T&I: ophthalmology, allergy, otolaryngology, dermatology, anesthesiology and pain medicine (n = 63, 14%).

5. Cluster 5 PSY: psychiatry, physical medicine and rehabilitation, preventive medicine and neurology (n = 45, 10%).

6. Cluster 6 DIAG: pathology, radiology, basic medical science, hematology, neuropathology (n = 48, 10%).

7. Cluster 7 OBGYN: obstetrics and gynecology (n = 27, 6%).

Data for each physician, collected at the time of admission to medical school, was obtained from the Longitudinal Study Database. Staff members of the Longitudinal Study developed, refined and introduced new data collection instruments throughout the course of the project. The first instruments to be administered were the Myers-Briggs Type Indicator (MBTI)[25,26] and the 16 Personality Factor Questionnaire (16PF)[27,28] along with an initial version of a background questionnaire. At the same time, researchers collected MCAT scores, National Boards Parts I and II scores, measures of first and second year success and clerkship grades. In 1969 we introduced the Physician Ideology Questionnaire (PIQ) and the Student-Faculty Role Questionnaire (SFRQ) and in 1971 we introduced the Career Rating and Preference Inventory (CRAPI). Because different measures were introduced at different times, there were many cases with missing data at different time periods. Consequently, the number of cases suitable for analysis differed for the different instruments and different scales. The number of cases used in the analyses were as follows: background information (n = 409), personality test scores (n = 344-430); PIQ (n = 339); SFRQ (n = 337); performance measures (n = 345-349); and career ratings (n = 168-210).

The first set of analyses that were run on the data were what I term "salience analyses" since they determine if the scores for a subgroup "stand out" when compared to the distribution of scores of the total group. Salience Analysis compares the dependent continuous variable scores for a single category within a set of categories to the scores on that continuous variable for the total set of categories by drawing independent random samples from the total set of scores. My version of this Monte Carlo technique is manifested in a computer program called *Random Sampler*[29]. For each category, the program draws 100 or more random samples, of a size determined by the sample size of the particular category, from the full set of scores (over all categories) on the dependent variable. It computes the mean, variance, median and mode of each random sample and then calculates the percentages of those measures that fall above or below the comparable measures obtained for the particular category. (The values for means are the only ones reported in this document). The probability that the category mean is different from the mean of the full sample is given by the proportion of sampled means smaller or larger than that observed for the category. Thus, if 95% of the randomly obtained means fall above that obtained for the category of interest and 5% fall below that value, the difference is considered significant at the 0.05 probability level. No assumptions about the form of the score distribution of the dependent variable are necessary.

For the Myers-Briggs Type Indicator, Psychological Types and combinations of Type sub-categories, the prediction situation is that of categorical-to-categorical prediction. This was accomplished by computing Chi Square values and their probabilities using another computer program I wrote specifically to generate Selection Ratio Type Tables for the MBTI[30]. The total sample was compared to two national samples in order to test for any bias in personality representativeness. For individual specialty clusters, the type table for the specialty cluster was compared to the type table for the remainder of the sample.

Results for Specialty Clusters

Note: probability levels (or percent of random sample means over or under that of the target category) are shown in parentheses following the finding.

The results of the Selection Ratio Type Table Analyses indicated that significantly more INTJ (.000), INFP

(.004), INTP (.000), ENTP (.001) and ENTJ (.000) Psychological Types applied to and/or were selected into UNM than would be expected on the basis of McCaulley's sample[31]. These are the types of students that typically "look good on paper" and present themselves well in interviews. Also, UNM received significantly fewer applications from and/or selected fewer ISTJ (.047), ISFJ (.003), ESFP (.005) and ESFJ (.000) Psychological Types. These are the types of students who may present themselves as humble and less sophisticated, are more practical than theoretical, and prefer hands-on, experiential learning over "book-learning." Results were the same for the CAPT sample[32] with the exception that UNM selected fewer INFJs than appeared in that sample (.005).

Internal Medicine Cluster

Physicians who eventually chose Internal Medicine or one of its sub-specialties as their medical specialty, upon entry to medical school rated as less desirable than their peers the specialties of General Practice (.02), Family Medicine (.00), Obstetrics-gynecology (.03) and Physical Medicine and Rehabilitation (.02). Their inclinations toward Internal Medicine (.01) and two sub-specialties, Allergy (.02) and Pulmonary Medicine (.01), were significantly stronger than that of their peers. Their academic interests were evident in higher levels of preference for working in a research facility (.00) and an educational institution (.00), the percent of professional time they wished to devote to research (.05), the importance of having a part-time affiliation with a medical school (.00) (and not living too far away from one (.03)), and being close to prominent persons in their field (.03). They wanted to work with other physicians (.02), and be free to try out their own ideas (.00) and mold their own roles (.01). Both personal characteristics (.00) and professional abilities (.04) of co-workers were important to them. They preferred working in a non-governmental facility (.01) and being able to control both their income (.04) and patient load (.03).

Choosers of the Internal Medicine Cluster did not distinguish themselves by their grade point average or their scores on any of the scales of the Medical College Admissions Test (MCAT). They were less likely than their peers to have had any prior work experience in a medical setting (.00).

On the 16PF, members of the Internal Medicine Cluster scored significantly higher on the Ego Strength Scale (.00), i. e., they tended to be less easily upset and more emotionally stable than their peers. On the Myers-Briggs Type Indicator, they were more likely to fall into the ESTJ Psychological Type (.038). According to the manual, ESTJs " live by a set of clear standards and beliefs, make a systematic effort to follow these, and expect the same of others. They value competence, efficiency, and results..." ESTJs are described as logical, analytical, and objectively critical, decisive, clear, well organized, and assertive. If they neglect their intuitive and feeling sides too much, they run the risk of becoming inflexible and dogmatic, running roughshod over others and refusing to listen. Consistent with the over- selection of this type for members of the Internal Medicine Cluster, these medical students were less likely to have IS (.004), IF (.020) or SP (.021) two-point codes on the MBTI.

On the Student-Faculty Role Questionnaire (SFRQ), the members of the Internal Medicine Cluster also revealed their academic orientation and, possibly, their identification with medical school faculty. They scored higher on the Ideal Student Role Scale (.03), believing students should really invest themselves in course work, be enthusiastic about learning, show academic scholarship, and be orderly and productive. Their higher scores on the Academic vs Clinical Orientation Scale (.04) indicated they felt it was important to become good teachers, develop research skills and be theoretically oriented. They scored higher on the Faculty Professional Activity Scale (.04), believing faculty should be involved in research and various kinds of non-teaching professional affairs. As students, Internists scored higher on the Camaraderie Scale (.05), wanting faculty members to get to know them well, and include them in social and unofficial affairs. Scoring higher on the Student-Faculty Cooperation Scale (.02), they wanted faculty to be friendly, encouraging and supportive while also giving feedback about their performance and, for their part, they would seriously consider what faculty had to say and seek them out for informal discussions. Higher scores on the Psycho-social Orientation Scale (.00) showed their desire to learn about psychological, social, and cultural factors in so far as they play a role in medical practice but they also wanted to find purpose and meaning in their professional roles and learn to understand themselves as reflected in their scores on the Personal Development Scale (.00).

Consistent with these attitudes, the members of the Internal Medicine Cluster were hard-working and achieved results from their efforts in medical school, earning significantly higher scores on almost all sections of the National Boards Examinations, both Part 1 (Anatomy (, Physiology, Biochemistry, Pathology, Microbiology and Pharmacology) (all at .00) and Part 2 (Medicine (.00), Surgery (.01), OBGYN (.05), Pediatrics (.01) and Physical Medicine (.04)). They had higher Success Indexes for both year one (.01) and year two (.01) and higher ratings on Basic Science for both years one (.01) and two (.02). They achieved significantly higher clerkship ratings for Medicine (.00), Surgery (.00), Pediatrics (.00), Obstetrics-gynecology (.02), and Psychiatry (.00). With respect to academic performance, members of this cluster stood out from all the other specialty clusters.

Surgery Cluster

At the time they entered medical school, doctors who eventually chose Surgery as a medical specialty showed a greater inclination than their peers toward nearly all of the surgery sub-specialties: Neurosurgery (.03), Orthopedic Surgery (.00), Plastic Surgery (.04), Thoracic Surgery (.01) and Otolaryngology (.00) as well as Gastroenterology (.01), and Physical Medicine and Rehabilitation (.00). While they did not want a highly specialized practice, they were less inclined than their peers toward the practice of Family Medicine (.02) and did not care to work for the Public Health Service (.02). Community size was of greater importance to them than to their peers in choosing where to practice (.01) and they did not want to do so in a small town or rural area (.02) nor did they want to live in a community with a "mixed" political climate (.01). It was not important to them how far they lived from a metropolitan area (.02), perhaps because they planned on living in a larger community. Consistent with surgeons' reputed valuing of "endurance," they discounted the importance of being able to control patient load (.04), number of work hours (.05) or of being able to mold one's own role in one's work-setting (.02). It was more important for them to work with other physicians (.03) but they were unconcerned about the personal characteristics of those with whom they worked (.00). For some reason, they did not show as much of an inclination to work with adults (.01) as did their peers but they wanted to devote a greater portion of their work time to research (.00).

Members of this cluster tended to have a greater number of siblings than their peers (.01) and they ranked UNM higher than other medical schools to which they applied (.01). They did not distinguish themselves by their scores on the MCAT scales or their GPA.

On the 16PF, surgery choosers scored higher on the Self-sentiment Scale (.04) (more controlled, self-disciplined and socially precise) and the Imaginative Scale (.05) (imaginative, wrapped up in inner desires, as opposed to practical, conventional). They tended to score lower on the Shrewdness Scale (.03) (more unpretentious, less socially aware). On the Myers-Briggs Type Indicator, they scored significantly lower on the TF Scale (.02) (more toward the tough-minded thinking or analytical end of the scale).

On the Student-Faculty Role Questionnaire, members of the Surgery Cluster scored higher on the Academic Orientation Scale (.01), considering it important to be theoretically oriented, develop their research skills and learn how to be good teachers. Scores on the Psycho-social Orientation Scale (.01) and the Personal Development Scale (.00) indicated they did not consider it important to learn about psycho-socio-cultural aspects of medicine nor to learn about themselves, find purpose and meaning in their professional roles or appreciate the beauty in life. On the Faculty Respectfulness Scale (.04), they did not find it important for faculty to be considerate of patients or students or to be a "good example" to students. Their lower scores on the Faculty Accommodation Scale (.03) the Faculty Openness Scale (.01) and the Recognition Scale (.02) suggested they were less inclined to want faculty to accommodate to student needs, to be open with students about what was happening behind the scenes in the medical school, or for students to receive recognition for their accomplishments or to be understood and appreciated as individuals. Overall, they appear to be highly self-reliant and deny needs for any kind of nurturance from faculty. On the Physician Ideology Questionnaire, the surgeons scored higher on the Disease Orientation Scale than did their peers (.00) viewing it as important for the physician to focus his efforts on the treatment of biological disease rather than becoming involved in preventive and psycho-social medicine.

The surgeons scored lower on the first year Success Index (.01) and Basic Science rating (.00). They also achieved lower scores on the National Boards, Part 1, Pharmacology Section (.05). Otherwise, their performance scores were not significantly different from random samples of scores.

Family Medicine Cluster

Upon entry to medical school, doctors who eventually chose to practice in the Family Medicine Cluster gave higher ratings than their peers to their inclinations toward Family Practice (.00), General Practice (.00) or Pediatrics (.01) as specialties. They were more drawn to Public Health (.00) and work for the Public Health Service (.01) than their peers. They were relatively less inclined toward Neurology (.00), Neurosurgery (.00), Pathology (.03), Psychiatry (.02) or Surgery in general (.00). They wanted to devote more work-time to administrative duties (.02) and a smaller portion to research (.02), being also less inclined to want to work in a research facility (.05). They indicated a greater desire to work in a county, state or city health department (.02), a greater desire to work in a government health program (.03) and less desire to work in an educational environment (.03) or a non-governmental agency (.00). They had a greater desire to work with the neonate population (.03), to practice alone (.05) in a moderately specialized practice (.00) (but not a truly generalized practice (.00)). Their practice community preferences were relatively well-defined: they wanted to practice in a small town (.02) or rural area (.00) and distance from a metropolitan area was not of concern to them (.01) nor was the desire to control type of patients (.04). They did not want to live in a "fast-paced" community (.00) nor one that boasted a wealthy (.02) or moderate (.00) average income. The ethnic distribution of the community they chose was important to them (.01) and they desired a community with a mixed political climate (.00). They had less inclination to live in the Mid-West (.00) and more inclination to live in the Rocky Mountain region (.03).

Twenty four percent of Family Medicine Cluster members were from small towns while 45% of students from small towns became members of the Family Medicine Cluster. They had lower average GPA scores (.01) than their peers and scored lower on the Verbal (.02) and Quantitative (.04) MCAT Scales.

Members of this cluster were over-selected (compared to the overall distribution of students who entered this medical school) into the INFJ (.030), ESTP (.017), and ESFP (.017) Psychological Types and the ES_P Jungian Type (.001). INFJs are a "counseling" type gifted with insight into human relationships and empathic understanding of the feelings and motivations of others. ESTPs focus on the here-and-now and take a pragmatic and action-oriented, energetic approach to problem solving, focusing on immediate results. At their best, they develop easy methods to do difficult things, are flexible, inventive, and resourceful, and are good team members. ESFPs are pragmatic and action- oriented, like the ESTPs, but they focus on meeting human needs in creative ways. They are described as warm, sympathetic, and tactful. Thus, this specialty cluster draws on several different types of people who can wield their respective talents with differing styles, all within the domain of Family Medicine. Members of this cluster were also more likely to have higher IS (.016) and ES (.009) two- point MBTI codes.

As might be expected from their specialty choice, members of this cluster averaged higher scores on the Psychosocial Orientation Scale (.00) of the Student-Faculty Role Questionnaire (i. e., the value placed upon learning about psychological, social, and cultural factors in so far as they are relevant to patient care and augment clinical ability). However, they had significantly lower scores on the Academic Orientation (.00), Faculty Accommodation (.01), Student-Faculty Cooperation (.04) and Faculty Openness Scales (.00), i. e., they did not subscribe to the idea that students should be extra hard-working and scholarly as opposed to developing clinical skills and experience; they did not want to develop informal relations with faculty nor have them accommodate to student desires or have them share issues of conflict in the medical school with them. They also preferred a more relaxed approach to medical education. On the Physician Ideology Questionnaire, Family Medicine Cluster subjects scored significantly higher on the Physician Authority Scale (.05) (importance for the physician to have control over his work setting and all aspects of patient care).

On the performance measures, members of this cluster scored less well than their peers on many criteria: Lower scores on the second year Success Index (.02) and Basic Science rating (.00); Lower scores on National Boards, Part 1 Physiology (.02), Biochemistry (.02) and Pathology (.04) Scales; Lower clerkship ratings for Medicine (.00) and Obstetrics-gynecology (.01); and lower scores on National Boards, Part 2 Medicine (.00), Surgery (.01), Obstetrics (.00) and Physical Medicine (.02) Sections.

Technique & Instrument Oriented Specialties

When looking ahead toward their future career in medicine, members of the T&I Cluster had fairly definite ideas about what features they wanted (or didn't want) in their practice. They were significantly less inclined than their peers toward Family Medicine (.03), General Practice (.00), Internal Medicine (.03), Gastroenterology (.02), Psychiatry (.04) and Public Health (.03) as specialty choices and more inclined toward Ophthalmology (.00) and Otolaryngology (.05). They did not want to work in a city, county or state hospital (.02) or health department (.00) or in a government health program (01) or government agency (.00) (including the military (.01), the Public Health Service (.00) or the VA (.01)). They did not want to work in a research facility (.01) but were more inclined than their peers to want to work in a hospital (.02) or large group practice (.01) setting. In constructing their careers they placed greater importance on the need to meet emergencies (.02), the type of patients they would work with (05), and their opportunity to work with a treatment team (.01). They placed less importance on working in a highly specialized specialty (.00) (sub-specialty) or being close to prominent persons in their field of medicine (.02), did not want to work with neonates (.02) or geriatric (.02) patients as much as did their peers and did not want to live in a community where the population was skewed toward older age groups (.00). They placed greater importance on pace of life (.04) when contemplating their practice community and wanted to work in a larger metropolitan area, not a small town (.00) or rural area (.01). They did not go along with the majority in wanting to live in the Rocky Mountain region (.01) and would consider employment in a foreign country (.03).

Members of the T&I Cluster had fewer girls in their family of origin (.01) compared to their peers and had higher Grade Point Averages (.04). However, they did not distinguish themselves in any way on any of the MCAT Scales.

On the MBTI, both ISTP (.000) and ESFJ (.003) Psychological Types were over-selected while ENTP Psychological Types (..035) were under-selected compared to the distribution of students that were accepted into this medical school. ISTPs are interested in how and why things work but find abstract theories uninteresting unless they can quickly apply them. When functioning at their best, ISTPs can sift through large amounts of data and move quickly to get to the core of a problem and solve it with the greatest efficiency and the least effort. ESFJs are described as warm, sympathetic, and helpful. They value security and stability, focus on the present and base their decisions on experience and facts. Though they enjoy variety, they adapt well to routine and don't like work that demands mastery of abstract ideas or impersonal analysis. Both ISTPs and ESFJs are practical and pragmatic. Members of this cluster were more likely to have the EJ two-point code (.039) and less likely to have the IF two-point code (.055), as one might expect from those types that were over-selected. T&I choosers scored lower on the 16PF Ego Strength Scale (.00) (more easily upset).

On the Student-Faculty Role Questionnaire, members of this cluster scored significantly lower on the Ideal Student Role (.03) and Faculty Respectfulness Scales (.04), i. e., they did not subscribe to the notion that students should be hard-working and faculty should respect patient (or student) needs. However, they considered it important, on the Psycho-social Orientation Scale (.00), that students learn about psychological, social, and cultural factors in so far as they are relevant to patient care and augment clinical ability. Their scores on the Personal Development Scale (.00) suggest they believe that students should find purpose and meaning in their professional roles, learn to understand themselves and the complexities of the world, and appreciate the beauty in life. Their scores on the Informal Relations Scale (.03) indicate they would like students to have informal contacts with faculty members, e. g., informal discussions, one-to-one talks, social affairs, office visits. The T&I choosers did not distinguish themselves from their peers on the Physician Ideology Questionnaire.

Members of this cluster achieved higher Success Indexes in both years 1 (.02) and 2 (.01) and higher scores on National Boards, Part 1, Biochemistry (02).

Psychiatry Cluster

Members of this cluster, as entry level medical students, were more inclined than their peers to choose Psychiatry as their specialty (.00) but they were also drawn to Family Medicine (.03), General Practice (.03) and Allergy (.05). They were not inclined to select Thoracic surgery (.02) as a specialty. Other than that, they had few defined features for their future careers. They wanted to work in a non- governmental facility (.01) but had not yet decided upon other characteristics of their desired practice organization. A community's political climate was important to them when choosing a place to practice (.02) and they wanted to work in a community with a fast pace of life (.00) where their spouse could gain employment or pursue a career (.00).

As children, 62% of the Psychiatry choosers lived in a large community from ages 14 to 18. They were less likely to have majored in a biological science as an undergraduate (.05) and more likely to have majored in a social science, the humanities or fine arts (.00). Their scores on GPA or any of the MCAT Scales did not distinguish them from their peers.

Psychiatrists scored lower on the 16PF Conservativism Scale (.02) (more experimenting, less respecting of traditional ideas), lower on the Ergic Tension Scale (.04) (more relaxed, less tense or driven), and higher on the Tender-minded Scale (.02) (more sensitive, less self-reliant, less tough- minded). On the MBTI this cluster was over-represented by INFJ (.024) and INFP (.001) Psychological Types, and less likely to be designated an E_TJ Jungian Type (.052), as one would expect. INFJs are the traditional "counseling" type personality with a natural bent toward understanding and appreciating human motivations and emotions. They are organized and decisive in implementing their objectives. INFPs are like INFJs in their natural empathic understanding of others but they are more adaptable, flexible and tolerant (unless some core value is threatened). Members of this cluster scored significantly higher on the SN Scale (.004) (more Intuitive), were more likely to have the NF (.003), NP (.002) and IN (.002) two-point codes and less likely to have the EJ (.016), SF (.013), and ES (.020) two-point codes. These results are generally consistent with the results of other studies of psychiatrists[66].

On the Student-Faculty Role Questionnaire Psychiatrists obtained significantly lower scores on the Personal Development Scale (.01) (the importance for students to find purpose and meaning in their professional roles, to learn to understand themselves and the complexities of the world, and to appreciate the beauty in life). Apparently, they feel that they have already attained those objectives or, at least, know the path to those ends. On the Physician Ideology Questionnaire, they obtained higher scores on the Biological Orientation Scale (.02) (the importance the respondent attaches to the physician's biological knowledge and skill in applying it) and lower scores on the Physician Authority Scale (.04) (the degree to which the respondent considers it important for the physician to have control over his work setting and all aspects of patient care). One would suspect that they have in mind a medication-oriented approach to treating mental illness.

Psychiatrists had higher ratings on their Basic Science performance for year 2 (.00) and they obtained higher scores on National Boards, Part 2, Psychiatry (01). However, their scores on Part 1 of National Boards for Anatomy (.03), Pathology (.02), and Pharmacology (.05) were lower than those for their peers.

Diagnostic Specialties Cluster

Members of the Diagnostic Cluster, as entry-level medical students, were more inclined to choose Pathology (.00) as a specialty and were not inclined toward Cardiology (.05). They did not want to have a solo private practice (.03) and preferred working in a structured setting such as the military (.03) or an independent foundation (.03). They had already decided on the type of work they wanted to do (.00), wanted to control their patient load (.02) and work hours (.01), and wanted to be able to try out their own ideas (.00). They were less inclined to want to work with children (.03) and wanted to devote a greater portion of their work time to supervision (.05) than did their peers. While the ethnic distribution of their practice community was important to them (.02), they did not want to practice in a poverty area (03).

Members of this cluster did not distinguish themselves on any background variables. They had significantly higher Grade Point Averages (.01) and scored higher on the MCAT Quantitative Scale (.03).

On the 16PF the diagnostic specialists scored higher on the Guilt Proneness Scale (.00) (more apprehensive, worrying and self-reproaching, less self-assured) and the Ergic Tension Scale (.05) (more tense and driven, less relaxed). They obtained lower scores on the Happy-Go-Lucky Scale (.05) (more serious, prudent, sober and less happy-go-lucky, less enthusiastic) and Venturesome Scale (.00) (more shy, and timid, less socially bold and spontaneous). One might suspect, from these scores, that these physicians chose these specialties that tend to have less direct and sustained patient contact in part to avoid arousing their anxieties and self-doubts. On the MBTI they had higher scores on the EI Scale (.00) (more Introverted).

On the Student-Faculty Role Questionnaire, members of this cluster had a more pronounced need for Structure (.03) in the educational enterprise (prompt feedback, specification of what is required, encouragement to ask questions, getting recognition, evaluation by means of regular tests) and a greater desire for Faculty Openness (.05) about issues of conflict within the school, revisions in school policy, what is expected of them. On the Physician Ideology Scale they obtained higher scores on the Physician Authority Scale (.03) (importance for the physician to have control over his work setting and all aspects of patient care).

Physicians in this cluster obtained higher scores than most of their peers on National Boards, Part 1, Microbiology (.02) and higher scores on National Boards, Part 2, Medicine (.03), Obstetrics- gynecology

(.03), Physical Medicine and Rehabilitation (.02) and Psychiatry (.05).

OBGYN cluster

Medical students who would later become obstetricians, when anticipating their future careers, distinguished themselves from their peers on relatively few features and primarily in terms of what they didn't want rather than in terms of their positive inclinations. They were disinclined toward Allergy (.01) as a specialty choice, disinclined toward group practice (.03) and particularly disliked mixed-specialty group practice (.00). They rated working with adolescents as less desirable than did their peers (.00) and were not drawn toward practicing in a politically liberal community (.04), even though they said that the political climate of their practice community was not important to them (.01).

Students in this cluster were younger in age than other students on admission to medical school (.05), had fewer boys (.02) and fewer siblings (.03) in their families of origin. Their father was less likely to be employed in a medical profession (.02) and had an occupational rank (Hollingshead Index) that was lower than that of their peers (.05). Compared to other schools to which they applied, their preference rank for UNM was higher than that of other students (.01). Their average GPA was lower than for other students (.05).

On the 16PF, future OBGYN physicians scored significantly higher than their peers on Superego Strength (.02) (rule-bound and conscientious as opposed to expedient, unrestrained) and Shrewdness (.00) (calculating, socially aware as opposed to unpretentious). They scored lower on the Openness Scale (.05) (toward the tough-minded rather than the tender-minded side). On the MBTI, OBGYN choosers scored more toward the Judging side of the JP Scale (.05) (more organized and planful). Superego Strength is correlated with Judging in this sample, so the two findings would be expected to support each other.

In terms of student-faculty roles, members of this cluster placed less emphasis on the importance of Informal Relations with faculty members (.05), e. g., informal discussions, one-to-one' talks, social affairs, office visits. They also scored lower on the Student-Faculty Camaraderie Scale (.01) (the importance of faculty being cheerful and humorous, getting to know students well, being included in social and unofficial affairs). On the Physician Ideology Questionnaire, the obstetricians scored higher on the Biological Orientation Scale (.00) (importance the respondent attaches to the physician's biological knowledge and skill in applying it). In short, they appear to be a no-nonsense group whose members want to focus only on what they consider to be important in medical education.

Members of this cluster had higher Clinical Science ratings than their peers in Year 1 (.02) but scored lower on National Boards, Part 1, Biochemistry (.00) and National Boards, Part 2, Medicine (.03).

Summary and Discussion

The UNM sample is biased more toward the intellectual-academic types than the practical, hands-on types in comparison with two national samples. During those early years of the medical school in New Mexico, some members of the admissions committee were criticized for trying to make the school a "Harvard on the Rio Grande" but they may have just been trying to ensure that a high percentage of their first graduating classes made it through the rigors of medical education by favoring those with good grades and high MCAT scores. While the bias may have implications for the generalization of the findings to other state medical schools, the relationships between specialty choice and antecedent variables found in this study can still be considered valid since all comparisons are between groups within the total sample. It should also be remembered that, when making a large number of comparisons on different variables, a certain proportion of them would be expected to turn out to be "significant" simply by chance (although we have no way of knowing which ones are the "chance results"). However, the number of significant associations identified in this study are orders of magnitude larger than what would be expected to occur simply by chance. If a finding does not seem to "make sense" within the context of the other findings, it may be one of those which occurred by chance. Henceforth, a summary and discussion of the results:

Members of the IM Cluster were aware of their attraction to internal medicine and some of its sub-specialties and avoidance of more general types of practice when they first entered medical school. They seemed to be attracted to the practice of medicine in an educational and research setting and preferred work-setting characteristics that would allow for such activities. They were not outstanding with respect to ability as measured by the MCAT or previous academic performance. However, their ESTJ personalities emphasized toughness, practicality, decisiveness, systemic thought and an orientation toward getting results. Although the over-representation of ESTJs for Internists has been found before[23], they are not the usual "academic types" typically found in studies using the MBTI (those are the INTJs and INTPs). ESTJs are more pragmatic and drawn to administrative and management positions while introverted intuitives, especially INTJs and INTPs are more inclined toward traditional scientific and technical areas, including academic pursuits. Thus, this sample of internists may represent an unusual sub-group of ESTJs. Their attitudes about medical education are consistent with getting things done: being hard-working, academically-oriented students who learn everything they are taught. The results of their efforts are revealed in outstanding performance ratings and scores on both parts of the National Boards.

Students who became surgeons were attracted to nearly all surgical sub-specialties from the very start. They were not attracted to Family Practice nor living in a small town. Their MCAT scores and GPAs were unremarkable. They were analytical and tough-minded, self-disciplined and unpretentious. Like the internists, they were academically oriented but they did not go for any of the nurturant aspects of medical practice and didn't want to receive any special treatment or accommodation to their own needs. They wanted to narrow their focus to the particular disease they were treating. Performance was mostly unremarkable except for their knowledge of basic science in the first year. The results do not support the claim that surgeons are extraverted or less rule-bound than other specialists but does support the idea that they are tough-minded[24].

Most members of the Family Practice Cluster knew their specialty preference from the start and also knew they did not want to become surgeons, pathologists or psychiatrists. They were not attracted to research or educational work but found work in a government facility or public health to be appealing. They found the fast pace of life in large towns to be aversive and wanted to practice in a small town in the Rocky Mountain Region. Many were themselves from small towns. They had no outstanding scores on any of the 16PF Scales, in contrast to the findings of Borges and Osmon[35] and Taber et al.[36] (who were trying to distinguishing between person-oriented and technique-oriented specialties). Three different Psychological Types were over-represented in this cluster: the counseling INFJ type, the practical-helper ESTP type and the warm and tactful ESFPs. Each type found Family Medicine to be compatible with their leanings and, apparently, family medicine had a place for all of them. Myers and Davis[37] found ESTJs to be the most common type in general practitioners in the 1950s while Friedman and Slatt, three decades later, found _SFJs to be over-represented. Taylor et al.[38] found family practice residents in 30 residency programs to be characterized by high Intuition (N) and Feeling (F) scores. Stilwell et al.[39] found physicians who chose primary care had high scores on *either* Introversion *or* Feeling. The present results suggest that at least three different types may be disposed to choose Family Practice and it may be that the proportions of these types differ slightly in the different research samples. The family practitioners in this sample liked the idea of learning about psychological, social and cultural factors in medical practice but were not academically minded. They did not want to fraternize with faculty or have them show them any special treatment. They were likely to have lower GPAs and MCAT Verbal and Quantitative scores and their second year and clerkship ratings were lower than those for their peers. They did less well than their peers on many scales of National Boards, Part 1 and Part 2.

As entering students, members of the Technique and Instrument Cluster were disinclined toward many specialties and attracted toward just two: Ophthalmology and Otolaryngology. They didn't want to work in any kind of government facility but liked hospitals and large group practices. They were attracted to work in large metropolitan areas and not in small towns or rural areas. Their MCAT scores were unremarkable but they had higher GPAs than their peers. The associations of technique-oriented physicians with Dominance, Vigilance and Tenseness on the 16PF found by Taber et al.[40] were not found in the current study. The practical ISTPs and ESFJs were over-represented while the more abstract ENTPs were under-represented. They did not subscribe to the notion that students should be studious and hard-working and desired to have informal contacts with faculty. They could see the value in learning about psycho-social medicine and developing their own personalities. Their medical school performance and scores on the National Boards examinations was about the same as their peers.

Members of the Psychiatry Cluster had been attracted to Family Medicine as well as Psychiatry when they entered medical school. Most features of their imagined medical practice were undefined except they wanted to live in a community with a fast pace of life and preferred non-government work settings. Most were from large cities and they were more likely to have majored in social science, the humanities or fine arts rather than a biological science. GPAs and MCAT scores were not significantly different from those of their peers. On the 16PF they were less conservative, more experimenting and free-thinking than their peers while also being more sensitive and relaxed. INFJ and INFP Psychological Types were over-represented. This is consistent with MBTI folklore and with the findings of Myers and Davis. However, Yang et al.[41] found no significant differences in the probability of students matching to psychiatry residency programs as a function of differences on the four basic contrasts of the test. They did not do any more sophisticated statistical tests but they did note that most of their psychiatry sample were higher on I, N and J than their opposites. In the present sample, Psychiatry choosers as entering medical students, did not find it necessary to work on their own self- development; they considered the physician's biological knowledge to be important but not his control of all aspects of medical care. Their scores on three sections of the National Boards, Part 1 were lower than that of their peers but they scored higher on the Psychiatry section of Part 2.

As entering students, members of the Diagnostic Specialties Cluster were attracted to Pathology but not Cardiology. They preferred working in a structured setting and wanted to control their work demands and have an opportunity to try out their own ideas. They had higher GPAs than did their fellows and higher MCAT Quantitative scores. They were more introverted, apprehensive, driven, and sober than other students and less spontaneous. In medical school, they wanted more structure and did not want to be kept in the dark about issues of contention in the school. They felt the physician should have control over all aspects of patient care. They did better than most other students on both parts of the National Boards.

Members of the OBGYN Cluster seemed to know what they disliked but not what they liked when entering medical school. They were younger, had fewer siblings and their fathers had a lower occupational index than did the fathers of their classmates. They tended to have lower GPAs. They appeared to be conscientious, organized, socially aware and tough-minded. (The higher MBTI scores of obstetricians on S, T and J found by Friedman and Slatt[42] were not found in this sample). Members of this group were averse to fraternizing with faculty and seemed to focus on just what they considered to be important in medical education, i. e., biological knowledge. They obtained higher Clinical Science ratings in their first year but not thereafter and they were below their classmates on one section each of the two parts of the National Boards.

It may not be evident from reading the results for each specialty group but members of the different specialties appear to respond differently to the different data collection methods. That is, obstetricians have 4.4 times as many significant findings than expected by chance for the background information (p = .000); psychiatrists have 5.4 times more significant findings in the personality domain (p = .001), internists have 1.7 times more significant results in the performance measures (.001), and Technique and Instrument Specialists have 1.5 times more significant findings than expected on the Career Rating and Preference Inventory (p = .016) and two thirds fewer significant results than expected on the performance measures (p = .046). Neither the SFRQ nor PIQ showed any significant differences between groups (although surgeons, with 1.9 times as many significant results than expected on the SFRQ, were close to significance (p=0.06)). In a similar vein, Jeffe, et al.[43] observed that their six primary care categories did not share a uniform set of predictors.

What these differences mean cannot be determined from the data themselves. What I suspect is that one or more "method factors" may be influencing the participants. Method factors represent variance common to indicators from the same data source. Some people may have an affinity or an aversion toward one kind of assessment device rather than another. That is, observed scores may be affected by variance stemming from unmeasured response tendencies (e. g., the tendency to cast oneself in a favorable light or to have "test taking anxiety") and/or the valences of the items themselves (e. g., how they are phrased) rather than simply the constructs that one intends to assess. The observed relationships between variables of interest might be inflated or deflated by variance due to the assessment method in addition to the underlying variables of interest. The SFRQ and PIQ both have items that are phrased in the least abstract way, compared to personality questionnaires for example, and are most relevant to the students immediate concerns and past experience. Students are experienced at being students and assessing the educational environment, having accumulated more than the required 10,000 hours to be considered "experts." Therefore, the SFRQ and PIQ may elicit less negative response bias than the other measures. Psychiatrists may be less defensive about inquiries related to personal matters and therefore be more willing to reveal themselves on personality measures. Whatever it is that is going on here, it is likely to make creating simple linear combinations of variables to predict outcome variables more difficult. In fact, devising linear combinations of variables is probably only a rough means of getting at the true relationships involved.

How well can students predict their specialty choice?

Do entering medical students have any inkling of the kind of medical specialty they might choose? Kassebaum and Szenas[44] reported that overall only 20% of the 12,753 students they studied maintained their specialty choice from beginning to end of medical school when simply asked to declare their intentions. "Generalist" specialties were more likely to endure but still this was for only 33.5% of those who made that kind of declaration. Jones et al.[45] found that, for all years in medical school, student predictions of what specialties they would *not* select was highly predictive of actually *not* selecting postgraduate training in those specialties. Positive predictions, however, did not fare so well until year three (except for family medicine which boasted of a 60% concordance rate in years one and two). Looney et al.[46] also found that they were able to predict who would *not* choose a generalized practice and rural area but not who would choose them. Scott et al.[47], using the selection of residency programs in Canadian medical students as the criterion, found a 60% concordance rate with entry level declaration of a specialty intention for pediatric choosers; 52% for family medicine choosers; 49% for internal medicine choosers; and 43% for surgery choosers. But psychiatry and obstetrics-gynecology choosers only showed 24% and 28% concordance rates, respectively. Compton et al.[48] found that only 30% of those students in 15 different medical schools who were interested in primary care on entry maintained that interest as compared to 68% for those interested in other kinds of specialties.

Methods

The present analysis used 187 student ratings of 10 specialty preferences (or dis-preferences) at the time they entered medical school to predict their actual memberships in one of seven specialty clusters at the end of their careers, instead of comparing a single declared specialty preference or a top ranked specialty with the specialty (or specialty training program) they eventually chose. It is believed that a set of specialty preference ratings is a more sensitive indicator of students' career inclinations than a simple declaration of one from an array of options because it incorporates more facets of the students' career dispositions. The bipolar nature of the scales incorporates both positive and negative inclinations toward alternative specialties into the subject's prediction, making it into an array variable.

In order to assess students' ability to anticipate their future careers, multiple discriminant function analyses were performed on sets of career ratings in relation to each dependent categorical variable. This procedure calculates a set of *discriminant functions,* linear combinations of variables somewhat like a regression equation only the objective is not to predict values on a continuous dependent variable but to separate the groups as much as possible. The procedure provides the number of correct and incorrect placements for each alternative category using those discriminant functions based on sets of predictor variables (in this case, preference ratings for those aspects of career).

Results

The Multiple Discriminant Analysis on the 10 specialty preference ratings and 7 specialty clusters produced two discriminant functions that significantly separated the specialty groups and an additional four functions that were not significant (Table 1).

Table 1. Discriminant Functions Extracted for Entry Level Specialty Preferences

No.	Root	Proportion	Canonical R	Chi-Squared	D.F.	Prob.
1	0.2800	0.4216	0.4655	106.7005	60	0.000
2	0.1856	0.2829	0.3957	63.3597	45	0.037
3	0.1097	0.1672	0.3144	33.1407	32	0.411
4	0.0499	0.0760	0.2179	14.6617	21	0.840
5	0.0242	0.0369	0.1538	38.3393	12	0.915
6	0.0100	0.0153	0.0997	1.7727	5	0.880

The predicted specialty group vs actual specialty group concordances appear in Table 2. The overall concordance rate (percent of correct placements) is 47%. Best prediction was for the Family Medicine Cluster (80%) while the poorest prediction was for the Psychiatry Cluster (19%).

Thus, it appears that only students who were inclined toward Family Medicine, on entry to medical school, had a pretty good idea that they would end up practicing in that field and that most of the others had, at best, only a little better than chance expectation of their eventual specialty choice.

In order to assess whether or not student predictions increased in accuracy over time in medical school, Multiple Discrimination Function Analyses were performed on student ratings of the same set of specialties for each year of medical school. The results appear in Table 3. As can be seen in that table, the predictability of Family Medicine remained rather high and constant up until the final two years of medical school, where it declined slightly. The predictability of membership in the Internal Medicine

Cluster increased in the last two years. The final year of medical school, after all clerkships were completed, saw an increase in the predictability of membership in all of the specialty clusters except for the Diagnostic Cluster.

Table 2. Classification Table for Predicted and Actual Specialty Group

Actual Group	Predicted Group						
	1 IM	2 SURG	3 FM	4 T&I	5 PSY	6 DIAG	7 OB
1 IM	9 (26%)	0	20	5	1	0	0
2 SURG	4	6 (32%)	7	1	1	0	0
3 FM	5	2	53 (80%)	4	0	2	0
4 T&I	3	2	8	10 (42%)	1	0	0
5 PSY	3	1	9	0	3 (19%)	0	0
6 DIAG	3	1	11	1	0	4 (20%)	0
7 OB	2	0	5	0	0	0	2 (29%)
Total	29	12	113	21	6	6	0

One-way analyses of variance between groups for the specialty ratings during year 4 generated significant F statistics at the following probability levels: Family Medicine (.000); General Practice (.001); Internal Medicine (.002); Obstetrics-gynecology (.004); Ophthalmology (.044); Orthopedics (.008); Otolaryngology (.037); Pediatrics (.000); Psychiatry (.001); and Public Health (.008). Fewer ratings generated significant F statistics in earlier years.

Table 3. Summary Table of MDF Analyses by Year of Medical School

	Entry	Year 1	Year 2	Year 3	Year 4
N	187	190	186	139	100
# Significant Anovas	4	3	3	5	10
# Significant Functions	2	1	2	2	4
Canonical R	0.47	0.42	0.45	0.56	0.71
% Correct IM	26	38	16	63	59
% Correct SURG	32	16	33	27	56
% Correct FM	80	83	82	74	69
% Correct T&I	42	23	25	35	72

% Correct PSY	19	14	22	36	69
% Correct DIAG	20	20	36	7	17
% Correct OB	29	0	17	9	63
Overall %	47	42	46	45	63

Another window on the specialty selection process is afforded by the seven-point bipolar rating scales: the changes in number of specialties rated as neutral, positive or negative over time in medical school can be assessed. A chart of these ratings at five different time periods appears in Figure 1. It can be seen from that diagram that number of negative ratings increase gradually over time while the number of specialties rated neutral decrease and the number of positives remain relatively constant. A two-way analysis of variance produced an F value of 129.017 with 2 degrees of freedom (p=0.000) for the valence of rating effect (neutrals, positives, negatives) and an F of 11.720 with 8 degrees of freedom (p=0.000) for the interaction effect (valence by year). Year by itself was not significant because of the divergence of neutral and negative ratings canceling each other out.

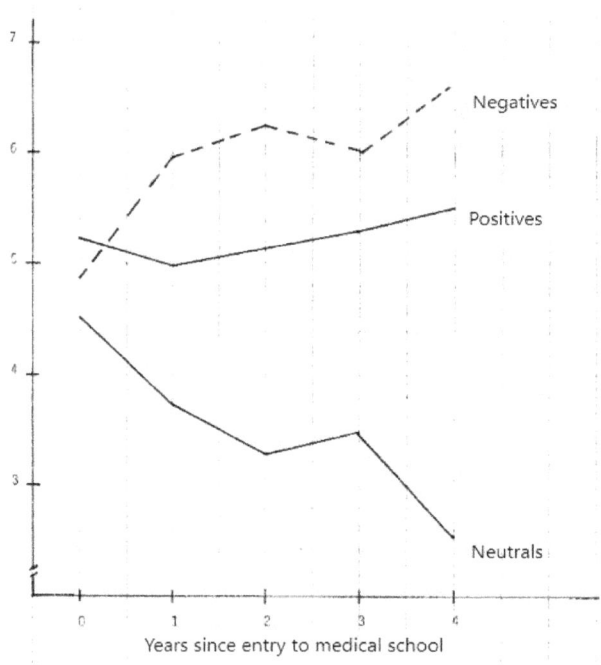

Figure 1. Number of positive, negative and neutral preferences during medical school.

The plots of response valence by year were basically the same for each of the specialty clusters except for the Surgical Cluster. The neutrals and negatives for surgeons diverged in the usual directions, as with the other clusters, but their number of positives were not significantly different from their negatives. Thus, what appears to be happening is that students are weeding out specialty options from the neutral category and placing them into the negative category, and to a lesser degree, in the positive category as they go along in medical school. The largest effect occurs in years 3 and 4 as students get direct exposure to different specialty milieus during their clerkship rotations.

Conclusions

Medical students who eventually choose a specialty within the Family Medicine Cluster are the only group of students to anticipate their eventual specialty with a high degree of accuracy from the time they are admitted to medical school. Internal Medicine choosers achieve a high degree of predictability in their third year of medical school while choosers of other specialties do not achieve a comparable level of predictability until they have completed medical school (or even later, in the case of the diagnostic specialties). Students appear to progressively weed out specialties from consideration as they go through medical school and develop more knowledge of the features of the different fields in medicine. Direct experiences during the clerkship years have the greatest effect on solidifying specialty preferences into specialty choices.

The results of this study suggest that 65% or so of students would not be able to declare a specialty intention with sufficient accuracy to enter a specialty track early in medical school. Except for those with intentions to enter a specialty in the Family Medicine Cluster, it appears that direct experience with the nuts-and-bolts of the specialties is needed to help students sort themselves into the different specialties. In situ learning experiences such as those provided by the MECO (Medical Education and Community Orientation) preceptorship programs implemented by the American Medical Student Association back in the 1970s have demonstrated that personal experience in certain kinds of medical settings can help undergraduate medical students clarify their career goals, including their choice of family medicine as a specialty[49]. Whether or not it would be feasible to develop similar programs for other specialty areas (such as psychiatry, which apparently is currently in need of recruits) is a question medical schools would have to determine, but it certainly seems possible.

On the other hand, most of the the 35% or so of medical students headed toward eventual practice in family medicine could be taken at their word (or, to be more accurate, their ratings of preference for several specialties) when they first enter medical school. They could be placed in tracks with a narrower focus than the ordinary medical school curriculum so as to speed their entry into an appropriate residency program. External preceptorships along the way might be provided to help reduce the amount of defection from their initial specialty goals and reinforce their efforts.

Addendum: Attitudes of Medical School Faculty as a Function of Departmental Affiliation

All full-time faculty members and clinical associates at the University of New Mexico School of Medicine, faculty who taught the students studied in the analyses shown above, were asked to respond to the items of the Physician Ideology Questionnaire, (PIQ) and the Student-Faculty Role Questionnaire (SFRQ) and to a biographical inventory. Of the 171 faculty members (43%) who responded to the biographical inventory, 21 (12.3%) were full professors, 20 (11.7%) were associate professors, 45 (26.3%) were assistant professors, 66 (38.6%) were clinical associates and 19 (11.1%) were instructors or lecturers. By professional character, they were: MD's 125 (73.1%); Biological Scientists (PhD's) 21 (12.3%); Social Scientists (including 10 (5.8%) clinical psychologists); Nurses, Social Workers and other allied health professionals 9 (5.3%); Librarians and laboratory professionals 4 (2.3%); and no response 2 (1.2%)

Respondents represented all 16 departments in the medical school, and had a mean age of 42 years. For most (55%), it was their first academic position.

Results

Eighty three of the pair-wise comparisons between departments produced t-values significant at or beyond the .05 level of confidence. Rather than describe all of the significant paired comparisons, the salient features of each specialty group will be indicated.

Psychiatry department faculty members were distinguished, on the PIQ, by strong inclinations to have the nurse take greater responsibility (relative to the physician) in the mutual exchange of information with patients and for controlling patient behavior (seeing that patients follow instructions, calming disturbed patients, clarifying hospital regulations). This probably reflects an egalitarian, role-sharing orientation toward nurses, rather than any desire to avoid dealing with such matters. They are strongly oriented toward psychosocial aspects of medicine and the lowest of the groups on the importance attributed to the physician's biological knowledge. They are more oriented toward community service and the use of community agencies than members of Medicine and Surgery departments. Their ideal physician would be much less concerned about his authority than would the ideal physician of the other departments.

Compared to faculty in other departments, psychiatry faculty members place the most value on teaching medical students about psychosocial aspects of medicine, perceive the least amount of such emphasis, and are most dissatisfied with this aspect of the curriculum. They hold the highest expectations for faculty members helping students to understand themselves and work out their problems, perceive fewer faculty members understanding students as individuals and being helpful and supportive toward them and are the most dissatisfied of all departmental groups with faculty performance in this respect. Compared to the other departments, they perceive fewer faculty members as efficient, well-organized and considerate teachers; perceive less openness with students about school policy and issues of conflict within the school; and perceive faculty members as less considerate toward patients. In addition, members of this department desire the most student influence in the determination of the educational process, perceive the least and would apparently like to see more than what they consider exists. Psychiatry faculty are also more dissatisfied with the amount of both student and faculty participation in extracurricular affairs. They see more emphasis on the development of clinical generalists than they expected.

The Department of Surgery appears, on the measures used here, to be the mirror-image of Psychiatry. The correlation between means for the two departments were -.65 for the PIQ scales, -.97 for SFRQ- 1; -.59 for SFRQ-2, and -.82 for SFRQ-3.

On the PIQ, surgeons saw less value in a psychosocial orientation in their ideal physician than the other clinical groups, placed the most importance on the physician's biological knowledge, were less community oriented than psychiatrists (but no more so than internists) and valued more than other groups the authority associated with being a physician. They were more prone than psychiatrists to state that it is the physician's responsibility to control patient behavior.

In their expectations of student-faculty relations, surgeons were the least psychosocially oriented, placed the least value on faculty acting in counselor roles with students and desired the greatest amount of faculty influence in the determination of the educational process of all groups. They perceived more student influence than other departments and more than they themselves desired. They grouped with members of Medicine and basic science in their relative (to Psychiatry) satisfaction with the amount of faculty helpfulness and support perceived to be given to students. Surgeons were the most satisfied with the amount of psychosocial emphasis in the curriculum, desired more emphasis on specialization and were relatively satisfied with the amount of student and faculty extracurricular activity.

Of the five departmental groups, basic scientists tended to place the least value on psychosocial aspects of patient care compared to other groups, their ideal physician would be more likely to handle matters of patient behavior-control himself and to have a relatively large amount of authority in deciding about patient care. It is interesting that the basic scientists placed no more value on the physician's biological knowledge than did other groups.

Expectations of student-faculty relations for the basic scientists did not differ much from those of other departments. They placed less importance on teaching students about psychosocial medicine than psychiatrists but more than surgeons. They desired more faculty influence than psychiatrists and placed less value on faculty trying to help students understand themselves and being supportive toward them. They perceived more faculty supportive activity toward students and were satisfied with the extent of it. Basic scientists saw the most faculty openness with students, psychosocial emphasis and faculty considerateness to patients, but perceived the least amount of "ideal student role" behavior.

Members of the Department of Medicine tended to be oriented to the psychosocial aspects of patient care as were the members of Psychiatry. Compared to the psychiatrists, they prefer their ideal physician to have more biological knowledge but be less oriented to community service and the use of community agencies and personnel. His ideal physician would be less concerned with authority over patient care than the surgeon's, but more so than the psychiatrists.

Except for a few characteristics, Internal Medicine seems to be an average group in terms of expectations of student and faculty behavior and satisfaction with their current relationship. They see the most academic emphasis in the curriculum, tend to perceive more student influence than most faculty and perceive the greatest amount of student interest and enthusiasm in learning.

The Pediatrics group did not differ much from the Medicine group except in being less psychosocially oriented and perceiving less academic emphasis in the curriculum. Compared to surgeons, they are less concerned with the physician having a lot of authority, consider it more important that students learn psychosocial medicine, desire more supportive behavior on the part of faculty and want more student influence in the educational process (although they don't want as much student influence as do psychiatrists). The Pediatrics faculty appear to be in the middle range in terms of satisfaction-dissatisfaction with student faculty relations, although somewhat more discontent than Medicine faculty.

Discussion and Summary

It seems reasonable to assume that medical students make their specialty selections on the basis of some kind of comparison between what they believe themselves to be and their perceptions of the demands, requirements and opportunities of different specialties. This process may be mediated, at least in part, by an assessment of characteristics of representatives of the specialties and one's similarity to them or ability to work with them. For many, if not most medical students, experiences with faculty members provide the first real opportunity to make such assessments and comparisons. The "images" projected by faculty members become associated with the specialties they represent and, for the student, aid in differentiating his own professional identity. It might be argued, therefore, that personality, value, attitudinal and stylistic differences in specialists are functional aspects of the medical school environment and are necessary for the professional development of the student.

The research literature suggests that there is a fair amount of consensus on how different specialists are viewed. Zimny and Thale[50], using the Gough Adjective Checklist, studied specialty characterizations by 62 graduating medical students. Internists were noted to be intellectual while surgeons were seen as domineering, arrogant, aggressive, full of energy and very concerned with their own prestige. Pediatricians were described as warm, friendly and responsible, and psychiatrists were stereotypes as placid, self-concerned, compliant and emotionally uninvolved with others. Bruhn and Parsons[51] found pretty much the same picture for these specialists. The general practitioner, they found, was seen as people oriented, aggressive, energetic, likable and patient.

The results of the present study seem to support the stereotypes of these specialists (with a few exceptions) and indicate some things about the way they may interact with medical students. According to the measures used in this study, psychiatrists are psychosocially oriented, egalitarian, value community service but not biological knowledge, argue for understanding of students as individuals and criticize other faculty for their lack of openness, effectiveness as teachers, considerateness towards patients, etc. Surgeons are "just the opposite" of psychiatrists: anti-psychological, anti-community, authoritarian, biologically oriented and highly specialized. Basic scientists, like surgeons, are not concerned with psychological factors in health and disease and value authority. They are critical of students, but not faculty. Members of the Medicine faculty are both psychosocially and biologically oriented are neither authoritarian nor laissez-faire, tend to praise students and value academic performance. Pediatricians are psychosocially oriented, supportive and understanding of students and would like them to have more influence in the determination of the educational process.

Further research might focus more directly on how medical students use this kind of information in their consideration of different career alternatives and on how much importance it has in comparison with other determinants of specialty selection.

4 THE WAY THEY WERE: WORK-SETTINGS

Gerald D. Otis

The distribution of physicians across different practice types or work-settings has been one of the most rapidly changing demographics in the last few decades. By 2016 less than half of physicians had any ownership share in their practice, down from 53.2% in 2012[52]. Among non-government practitioners, solo practitioners dropped from more than 40% in 1983 to 16.5% in 2016. Single specialty group practice garnered 42.8%, down 2.7% from 2012, while mixed-specialty groups climbed to 24.6%[53]. In 2016 there were 32.8% of physicians working in hospitals as employees or in a hospital owned practice[54, 55]. Among those physicians under 45 years of age, only 3% were in solo practice while 28% were in medical groups: 18% (small group), 11% (mid-sized group) and 24% (large group). Hospitals captured 28% of these young physicians while medical schools employed 11%. Only 25% said they would choose the same practice setting again while 30% planned to change employers. (40% said they would not choose medicine as a career again)[56, 57].

Research on determinants of choice of practice work-setting has not garnered the same amount of attention as that for specialty choice. Most has focused on income optimization, economies of scale, time pressures and work-load characteristics, social orientations to medical practice, attitudes toward managerial and office tasks, and attitudes toward political influences on medical care. For primary care physicians, Ubokudom[58] found older physicians to be more likely to locate in affluent and under-served counties than group practitioners and female physicians were more likely to practice in institutional settings. One interesting study[59] looked at the differences in the potential for "peer regulation" between solo, small group and large group practices, taking into account environmental characteristics of the community, sociodemographic characteristics of the physicians and their attitudes toward such things as quality of patient care, the business side of practice, scheduling predictability, desire for personal autonomy and income potential.

Perhaps the most ambitious effort to define physician work-settings was the project by Quenk and

Albert [60] as part of the UNM Longitudinal Study. Using a random sample of physicians obtained from the AMA, they developed a questionnaire containing numerous items characteristic of different physician activities and sources of satisfaction or dissatisfaction. Subjecting responses to these items to factor analysis, they derived seven dimensions characterizing physician work-settings: personal patient involvement; physician-teacher role; personal control of one's professional situation; medical innovation; personal control of income; interaction with the medical community; and professional ambition. Scores on these factors were then subjected to typological analysis (object grouping) to derive seven "physician niches" to which the subjects belonged: technical specialist; traditional primary care; situational constraint; service institutional; traditional specialist; physician statesman; and medical teacher. When analyzed with respect to measures of satisfaction, it was found that the situational constraint members were least satisfied while the traditional specialists were most satisfied. Dissatisfaction was inevitably associated with low scores on the personal control of professional situation dimension. In another analysis of this data, reported below, Quenk[61] developed regression equations for predicting satisfaction with their careers for each of several different specialties and work-settings.

The present study investigates the associations between chosen work-setting of a group of end-of-career physicians and many features of these same physicians at the time they entered medical school nearly half a century earlier.

Methods

Work-settings were defined as follows: solo private practice (20%); solo with one or more hospital affiliations specified (8%); small group up to 10 members (16%); medium group with 11-99 members (8%); large group with 100 or more members (4%); hospital-based (25%); university environment (12%); and government facility (7%). It should be noted that members of the present sample had probably practiced in other types of work-settings earlier in their career. However, with the exception of large group practice, the order of percentages is not far from the national samples.

Subjects, data, and analytical procedures (salience analysis, treatment of MBTI data, and multiple discriminant function analysis) are all the same as those described in Part I.

Results of Salience Analysis for Selection of Work-Settings

Listed below are the results of salience analysis for each work-setting category. The number of cases for these analyses were: background (n = 353), personality (n = 353), SFRQ (n = 272); PIQ (n = 277); performance (n = 353), career ratings (n =185). Significance levels for the salience analyses appear in parentheses.

Solo Private Practice

When looking ahead toward their future careers, medical students who eventually chose solo private practice as their work setting wanted to devote more of their time, compared to their peers, to direct contact with patients (.01) and less time to program planning (.03), case consultation (.02), or professional community service (.03). They gave higher ratings to being able to control one's own role, duties and activities (.01) and considered it more important to be in a high demand/low supply specialty for the area (.03). They were less inclined to want to work in a county, state or city health department (.02), or to practice in a suburb (.04) or on the West Coast (.00). They preferred to practice in a community with a moderate average income (.01) and did not consider it important for their chosen community to have opportunities for their preferred recreational, cultural or entertainment activities (.01). They indicated that they spent less of their leisure time in individual or solitary activity (.01) or with friends (.02) than did their fellow medical students.

Solo practitioners were older than their peers upon admission to medical school (.03). Both parents had less educational attainment than the parents of their peers (.00, .03) and their fathers, who were less likely to be physicians (.02), had lower occupational levels (.03).

They were more likely to have lower GPAs than their peers (.03) and scored lower on the MCAT General Information (.00) and Science (.01) Scales.

Choosers of the solo private practice model scored lower on the 16PF Imaginative Scale (more practical and conventional) (.04) and the IQ Scale (more disposed to concrete rather than abstract thinking) (.03). They scored higher on the Outgoing Scale (warmhearted, easy-going) (.05) and the Emotionally Stable Scale (calm, not easily upset) (.05).

These students scored higher on the Academic Orientation Scale of the SFRQ (the importance of becoming a good teacher, being theoretically oriented, developing research skills; as opposed to the importance of becoming a good clinician, being practically oriented, and gaining experience working with patients) (.05) (which seems counter-intuitive, at first, but makes sense if it is understood as something they *should* do to overcome their natural laid-back disposition.

That they were unable to do so is revealed in their academic performance measures. They had lower Success Indexes (.00) and ratings on their performance in Basic Science (.00) during their first year and they had lower ratings for their OBGYN clerkship (.00). On National Boards, Part 1, they had lower scores on Anatomy (.04), Microbiology (.00), Pathology (.00), Pharmacology (.00), Physiology (.01) and Biochemistry (.00) sections. On Part 2 of National Boards they scored lower on the Medicine (.00), OBGYN (.00), Pediatrics (.01), Physical Medicine (.04) and Surgery (.02) sections.

Solo Private Practice Plus Hospital Affiliations

Choosers of this type of practice model wanted to spend more time than did their peers doing research (.04) and less time in direct patient care (.02) and administration (.04). They were less inclined to work with adolescents (.03) and did not care to work in a county, state or city hospital (.00) or health department (.00). They were less inclined to work in a government health program (.03) or in a non government institution or agency (.00). They were less disposed to working for the Public Health Service (.00) and did not care to practice in a community whose population is skewed to the older ages (.01). They were more inclined to practice in the South Central region of the US (.01) and did not consider distance from a metropolitan area to be important (.04). As students, they spent less of their leisure time in civic, church, political or other task-oriented groups (.05).

Solo Plus practitioners had more boys (.02) and fewer girls (.02) in their families of origin. Their fathers tended to have higher educational attainment that did the fathers of other medical students (.03).

On the 16PF these students scored lower on the Happy-Go-Lucky Scale (more sober, serious, taciturn) (.04), the Shrewdness Scale (more forthright, natural, sentimental) (.01), and the Emotionally Stable Scale (easily upset, more affected by their feelings) (.02). They Scored higher on the Tenseness Scale (driven, frustrated, fretful) (.00).

These students did not distinguish themselves by any of their scores on the SFRQ scales but did score lower on the Physician Authority Scale of the PIQ (i. e., they considered it less important for the physician to have control over his work setting and all aspects of patient care) (.02).

Solo Plus students had higher ratings for Basic Science (.02) and had higher Success Indexes (.02) for their first year than did their peers. They also achieved higher scores on Part 2, National Boards Psychiatry (.01) and Physical Medicine (.01) sections.

Small Group Practice (<=10)

Medical students who would eventually choose to work in a small group practice setting believed it was important to work in their preferred type of work setting (.02), which, at that time, was solo private practice (.04). They liked the idea of working with other physicians on some joint task (.00) and held that it was important to expand their knowledge in their area of medicine (.01). They did not think the political climate of their practice community was important (.00) and spent more of their leisure time, as students, in structured recreational groups than did their peers (00).

Small group practitioners had lower scores on the MCAT Quantitative Scale (.00).

Small group physicians were more likely to have turned out on the MBTI as an ENFJ Psychological Type (.013) and to have had the EJ two-point code (.028). ENFJs are warm, compassionate, loyal and trustworthy. They can see the potential in others and like to help them realize it. They can be persuasive and get groups of people involved in a project in a harmonious fashion.

These respondents obtained higher scores on the Physician Professional Activity Scale of the SFRQ (believing it was important for faculty to be involved in non-teaching professional affairs such as research, clinical work, community participation) (.02) and higher scores on the PIQ Disease Orientation Scale (i. e., they considered it important for the physician to focus his efforts on the treatment of biological disease rather than becoming involved in preventive and psycho-social medicine) (.00).

Small group practice choosers had lower clerkship ratings in Medicine (.00) and scored lower on National Boards, Part 2, Medicine (.01), OBGYN (.03), Pediatrics (.00), Physical Medicine (.00) and Psychiatry (.00) sections.

Medium-Sized Group Practice (11-69)

When contemplating their future careers, medical students who would end up practicing in a medium-sized group work-setting had already decided upon the type of work they wanted (clinical, research, etc.) (.00). They were more inclined to work with an adult population (.00) even though they wanted to live in a community with its population skewed toward the younger age group (.02). They found it less important to have a part-time affiliation with a medical school (.01) or to live near one (04). They wanted to devote a greater portion of their time to professional community service (.05), were less likely to desire working in a government health program (.03) or practicing in a foreign country (.03).

These respondents were younger than their peers when entering medical school (.00) but were more likely to be married (.02) and they had higher Grade Point Averages (.00).

Medium-sized choosers had lower scores on the 16PF Assertiveness Scale (mild, conforming, humble) (.00). On the MBTI they had scores more on the Introverted end of the EI Scale (.04) and more on the Feeling side of the TF Scale (.04). They were more likely to have an IP two-point code (.043), an SF two-point code (.011), and were more likely to fall into the ISFP Psychological Type (.001). ISFPs are quiet and unassuming, sensitive to the practical needs of others and gentle in dealing with them. They like nature, especially animals, and want to contribute to people's well-being in their work, often by engaging in day-to-day care-taking activities as opposed to more abstract psychological understanding.

On the SFRQ these individuals tended to score lower on the Personal Development Scale (the importance for students to find purpose and meaning in their professional roles, to learn to understand themselves and the complexities of the world, and to appreciate the beauty in life) (.05) and the Psychosocial Orientation Scale (the value placed upon learning about psychological, social, and cultural factors in so far as they are relevant to patient care and augment clinical ability) (.01).

These medium-sized group members had the most deviant PIQ scores of all practice setting types. They scored lower on Psychosocial Orientation (importance for the physician to have knowledge and skill in interpersonal relations and apply that knowledge and skill to the social and emotional problems of patients) (.04), Community Orientation (the degree to which they considered it important that the physician be involved in health-related community activities other than patient care) (.00), Biological Orientation (importance attached to the physician's biological knowledge and skill in applying it) (.02), and Division of Responsibility (the degree to which they thought the physician (rather than the nurse) should obtain information and provide information to the patient and his/her family) (.05). They scored higher on the Disease Orientation Scale (importance of the physician focusing his efforts on the treatment of biological disease rather than becoming involved in preventive and psycho-social medicine) (.02). So, it appears that these no-nonsense practitioners did not want to learn about any of the "warm and fuzzy stuff" in regard to patients or in regard to themselves. They didn't want to be bothered with psycho-social matters in their practice or be otherwise involved in their community. They simply wanted to concentrate on what they considered their core task of helping patients in practical ways.

Medium-sized group practice choosers obtained higher ratings than did their peers for Basic Science in both years 1 (.01) and 2 (.00), and higher ratings in Clinical Science in year 1 (.00). Their Success Index was higher than that of their peers in both years 1 (.00) and 2 (.00). On National Boards they scored higher on Part 1 Anatomy (.00), Microbiology (.03), Pathology (.00), Pharmacology (.00), Physiology (.00) and Biochemistry (.00) and on Part 2 Medicine (.04), Obgyn (.00) and Surgery (.01).

Large Group Practice (>100)

Anticipating their future medical careers, physicians who chose to work in a large group practice were less inclined toward working with adults (.00), less inclined toward selecting Family Practice as a specialty (.03) and more inclined to work in a county, state or city health department than were their peers (.02). They wanted to devote a greater portion of their work time to teaching (.02) and a lesser portion of time to case consultation (.02).

While both their fathers and mothers tended to have less educational attainment than did the fathers and mothers of their peers (.01, .01), their fathers were more likely to have been employed in a medical field (.01). Respondents in this category of practice model achieved higher GPAs (.03) than did their fellow students but they were not significantly different from randomly selected students in their performance on the MCAT.

On the 16PF, large group practitioners obtained higher scores on the Control Scale (socially precise, self-disciplined, compulsive) (.03), the Imaginative Scale (bohemian, less conventional, careless of practical matters) (.01), and on the Tender-mindedness Scale (sensitive, less self-reliant, more over-protected) (.01). They scored more toward the Feeling side of the Myers-Briggs Type Indicator TF Scale (more empathic, guided by personal values, compassionate, striving for harmony and positive interactions) (.01).

On the SFRQ, large group practitioners scored higher than their peers on the Informal Relations with Faculty Scale (desirous of informal contacts with faculty members, e. g., informal discussions, one-to-one' talks, social affairs, office visits) (.05) and the Psychosocial Orientation Scale (valued learning about psychological, social, and cultural factors in so far as they are relevant to patient care and augment clinical ability) (.01). They scored lower on the Division of Responsibility Scale (wanting more student influence in preparing educational materials, deciding what's important to learn, providing instruction, determining educational methods, choosing professional goals, specifying methods of study or learning, and in relations with administrative personnel) (.01). This group did not distinguish themselves from their peers on any of the Physician Ideology scales.

In terms of academic performance, they were different from other medical students in that they achieved higher Basic Science ratings in their second year (.03).

Hospital-based Practice

Medical students who would eventually choose to practice in a hospital were more inclined to work with children (.02), less inclined toward solo private practice (.02) and wanted to devote less of their work time to teaching than did their peers (.00). More than other students, they preferred practicing in a wealthy community (.03). As students, they said they spent more of their leisure time in unstructured outings with friends (.02) and in professional groups (.03).

Hospital practitioners tended to be younger (.03) on admission to medical school. They had higher scores on the MCAT General Information (.05) and Science (.04) Scales than their classmates.

These respondents scored higher on the 16PF Happy-Go-Lucky Scale (more cheerful and enthusiastic, less sober, less prudent, less serious) (.03), and lower on the Self-Sufficiency Scale (more group dependent, good followers) (.05). On the MBTI, they were significantly more likely to fall into the ISTP Psychological Type (.000). ISTPs are expedient and believe in doing only what is needed with the least possible discussion and fuss. They tend to resist regimentation and rules and like novelty and the challenge of solving problems with concrete, unemotional logic.

Hospital practitioners scored higher on the Student-Faculty Cooperation Scale of the SFRQ (the value attached to students being considerate of faculty yet making suggestions to them and seeking them out for informal discussions; and of faculty being friendly and supportive, encouraging and accommodating to students and giving them feedback concerning their performance) (.05). They obtained lower scores on the Division of Responsibility Scale (in the direction of more desired student influence) (.02). On the PIQ they were more likely to have higher scores than their peers on the Biological Orientation Scale (the importance attached to the physician's biological knowledge and his/her skill in applying it) (.01).

Hospital-based practitioners scored higher than randomly selected students on National Boards, Part 1 Pathology (.04) and Part 2 Medicine (.00), OBGYN (.01) and Surgery (.04) sections.

University-based Practice

Medical students who ended up working in university settings had their sights on such an outcome when they first entered medical school. More than other students, they indicated that working in their preferred work setting was important to them (.01) and this preferred setting was an educational institution (.01) (although an independent medical foundation (.02), a research facility (.03), a government health program (.02) might be able to substitute). They were more inclined to work in a private hospital (.03) or large group practice (.02) or a non-government facility (.02). They were more inclined to work for the Public Health Service (.04) or the VA (.01). It was important for them to have a variety of practice opportunities available (.01), to be near a medical school (.04), to control their income (.03) and to work with an adult population (.00). They wanted to devote a greater portion of their time to teaching (.00) and they were more inclined to stay in the Rocky Mountain Region (.00). As students, they spent less leisure time than did other students in unstructured outings with friends (.01).

Members of this type of practice did not distinguish themselves on any background measures but they did have higher scores on the MCAT General Information Scale (.02).

On the 16PF, university-based practitioners scored lower on the Happy-Go-Lucky Scale (more serious, prudent, sober, less enthusiastic) (.03), lower on the Guilt-Proneness Scale (more self assured, confident, placid, less worrying or apprehensive) (.04), and lower on the Venturesome Scale (more restrained, shy, timid as opposed to socially bold, spontaneous) (.00). They scored higher on the Self-Sentiment Integration Scale (more controlled, self-disciplined as opposed to casual, careless of protocol) (.00).

The only SFRQ scale this group scored higher on than their peers was the Traditional (Ideal) Student Role Scale (.05) that assesses the degree to which students should really invest themselves in the work of a course, seriously consider what faculty say, be enthusiastic about learning, show interest in course material, be punctual, show academic scholarship, be orderly and productive, etc. Perhaps they identified with this role prescription. One would have thought they would show outstanding scores on some of the other SFRQ scales (e. g., Academic Orientation, Teaching Efficiency, Structure or Recognition) but they did not. Perhaps their thinking had not yet progressed to some of the other roles that faculty are required to enact.

On the performance measures, university choosers had higher ratings in Clinical Science during the second year of medical school (.01) and obtained higher ratings from faculty for their clerkship performance in their Surgery rotation (.00). They obtained higher scores on National Boards, Part 1 Microbiology (.04) and Pharmacology (.02) and higher scores on Part 2 Pediatrics (.04), Physical Medicine (.01) and Psychiatry (.01).

Government Practice

As one might expect, medical students who eventually ended up working in government facilities showed greater inclination to work in a county, state or city hospital (.00) or health department (.03) but they denied that it was important to them to be able to work in their preferred work setting (.03). They had a greater inclination to work in a hospital setting (.01) with either a neonate (.02) or older (.01) population. However, they also were favorably inclined toward solo private practice (.05) but disinclined toward work in a large medical group (.05). It was not important to them how much "red tape" was involved in the job (.02). They wanted to devote a smaller portion of their time to teaching (.04), didn't consider it important to have variety in their work activities (.03) or to work with either other physicians (.00) or non-physicians (.02) on a joint task. They did prefer to practice in a wealthy community (.02).

Government practitioners were more likely to be married when they entered medical school (.02) but they were not distinguished by their GPAs or MCAT scores. The only personality measure they stood out on was the I_TP Jungian Type (.05) on the MBTI.

On the SFRQ those physicians who chose to work in a government facility scored lower on the Academic Orientation Scale (the importance of becoming a good teacher, being theoretically oriented, developing research skills; as opposed to the importance of becoming a good clinician, being practically oriented, and gaining experience working with patients) (.05) and the Professional Activity Scale (the importance attributed to faculty involvement in non- teaching professional affairs - community participation, research, clinical work, medical school affairs) (.00). They scored higher on the Faculty Respect Scale (consideration shown to patients during interviews and examinations, requesting their permission for procedures to be carried out, explaining procedures; also, the importance of faculty being "good examples" in their dealings with patients, being patient with students who don't understand, respecting individual student interests, etc.) (.02). On the PIQ these respondents scored lower on Disease Orientation (i. e., they favored involvement in preventive and psycho-social medicine over focusing on treatment of biological disease) (.03).

Government practitioners received lower Success Index Scores in year 2 (.03) and were rated lower on their Psychiatry clerkship (.02) but they received higher clerkship ratings in Medicine (.00) and OBGYN (.00). Their scores on the Surgery Section of National Boards Part 2 were also lower than that of their peers (.00).

One might expect that work-setting choice could be related to specialty choice. When cross-tabulated and subjected to chi square analysis, the overall table was not significantly different from a random model but three cells of the table were significantly different than expected: Family Medicine was over-represented in Solo Private Practice and under-represented in Solo Private Practice Plus with hospital affiliations; and OBGYN was over-represented in Small Group Practice (See Table 4). Otherwise, it appears that it is possible for any specialty to be in any kind of work-setting.

Table 4. Cross-tabulation of Work-Settings by Specialty Clusters

Specialty Cluster	Work Setting								Total
	Solo	Solo+	SmGrp	MedGrp	LgGrp	Hosp	Univ	Govt	
IM	3 (5.5)	4 (3.6)	3 (6.7)	4 (3.4)	1 (1.4)	9 (6.9)	9 (4.9)	3 (3.6)	36 (20%)
SURG	2 (2.6)	4 (1.7)	3 (3.2)	1 (1.6)	1 (0.7)	3 (3.2)	1 (2.3)	2 (1.7)	17 (9%)
FM	18 (10.3)**	1 (6.6)*	15 (12.5)	6 (6.3)	3 (2.6)	8 (12.9)	7 (9.2)	9 (6.6)	67 (37%)
T&I	1 (3.5)	3 (2.3)	5 (4.3)	4 (2.1)	1 (0.9)	6 (4.4)	2 (3.2)	1 (2.3)	23 (13%)
PSY	3 (2)	3 (1.3)	0 (2.4)	0 (1.2)	1 (0.5)	3 (2.5)	1 (1.8)	2 (1.3)	13 (7%)
DIAG	1 (2.9)	2 (1.9)	4 (3.5)	2 (1.8)	0 (0.7)	5 (3.7)	4 (2.6)	1 (1.9)	19 (10%)
OB	0 (1.1)	1 (0.7)	4 (1.3)**	0 (0.7)	0 (0.3)	1 (1.3)	1 (1)	0 (0.7)	7 (4%)
Total	28	18	34	17	7	35	25	18	182
Pct.	(15%)	10%	19%	9%	4%	19%	14%	10%	100%

Numbers in parentheses are expected values. * Significant at .05 level. ** Significant at .02 level.

Multiple Discriminant Function Analysis for Work-Settings

When Multiple Discriminant Function Analysis was performed on the work-setting categories, using as predictors the preference ratings that entry level students gave to 13 work-setting options plus measures relating to how they wished to allocate their work time (direct patient care, teaching, program planning, case consultation, community service, supervision or research), only one significant discriminant function was produced (see Table 5). The procedure was able to classify only 65% of the total cases (Table 6), i. e., 35% were not assigned to any category. Using the total number of cases as a base, the average number of correct classifications was only 33%. The best hit-rate was for government employment followed by solo plus and large group practice. The poorest prediction was for solo private practice, with only 21% correct classifications.

Table 5. Results of MDF Analysis for Work-Settings

No.	Root	Proportion	Canonical R	Chi-Squared	D.F.	Probabilities
1	0.6920	0.3468	0.6395	173.8324	140.0000	0.0280
2	0.4433	0.2222	0.5542	119.1385	114.0000	0.3520
3	0.3215	0.1612	0.4933	80.9766	90.0000	0.7410
4	0.2295	0.1150	0.4320	51.9812	68.0000	0.9250
5	0.1398	0.0701	0.3502	30.4956	48.0000	0.9770
6	0.0897	0.0449	0.2868	16.8886	30.0000	0.9740
7	0.0795	0.0399	0.2714	7.9588	14.0000	0.8910

Repetition of these analyses for each year of medical school did not improve the results to any degree.

Table 6. Classification Table for MDF Analysis on Work-Settings

Actual Group	Predicted Group								Total
	Solo	Solo+	SmGrp	MedGrp	LgGrp	Hosp	Univ	Govt	
Solo	6 (21%)	1	0	1	2	8	0	0	18/28
Solo+	1	8 (44%)	0	1	0	1	0	0	11/18
SmGrp	0	2	9 (26%)	0	1	7	0	1	20/34
MedGrp	1	0	0	4 (24%)	3	0	1	1	11/17
LgGrp	1	0	2	0	3 (43%)	0	0	0	6/7
Hosp	3	1	1	1	0	15 (43%)	0	0	27/35
Univ	0	1	2	0	0	0	6 (24%)	1	10/25
Govt	0	0	1	2	0	4	0	9 (50%)	16/18

| | Total | 12 | 13 | 15 | 09 | 06 | 39 | 9 | 16 | 119/182 |

Thinking the categories of work-settings might be too specific for entry-level students, the groups were further collapsed into three groups : Solo Private Practice(25%), Group Practice (32%) and Institutional Practice (43%). The breakdown by specialty appears in Table 7. Chi square analysis of work-setting by specialty again produced no significant results. That is, it cannot be said that specialty cluster and work-setting are significantly related, given the marginal probabilities.

Table 7. Cross-tabulation of Work-Settings by Specialty Cluster.

Specialty Cluster	Solo Practice	Group Practice	Institutional Practice	Total
1 IM	7 (9)	8 (11.5)	21 (15.5)	36 20%)
2 SURG	6 (4.3)	5 (5.4)	6 (7.3)	17 (9%)
3 FM	19 (16.8)	24 (21.4)	24 (28.8)	67 (37%)
4 T&I	4 (5.8)	10 (7.4)	9 (9.9)	23 (13%)
5 PSY	6 (3.3)	1 (4.2)	6 (5.6)	13 (7%)
6 DIAG	3 (4.8)	6 (6.1)	10 (8.2)	19 (10%)
7 OB	1 (1.8)	4 (2.2)	2 (3)	7 (4%)
Total	46 (25%)	58 (32%)	78 (43%)	182 100%

Note: Numbers in parentheses are expected values.

Multiple Discriminate Function Analysis on the three work-setting groupings using 9 work-setting preference ratings and percentages of effort desired to be devoted to 3 different areas of work (direct patient care, teaching and community service) resulted in one significant discriminant function (Table 8).

Table 8. Results of MDF Analysis on 3 Category Work-Setting Choices

No.	Root	Proportion	Canonical R	Chi-Squared	D.F.	Probabilities
1	0.1905	0.5733	0.4000	42.2123	24	0.0120
2	0.1418	0.4267	0.3524	18.2345	11	0.0760

The predicted by actual classification table is shown in Table 9. The overall percentage of correct placements was 56% with the best hit rate being for subjects who chose to work in hospitals or other institutions (76%). The poorest prediction was for solo private practitioners, who were misclassified as institutional practitioners 44% of the time. Group practitioners were misclassified as institutional practitioners 43% of the time. The discriminant functions appear to be biased most toward classifying subjects as institutional practitioners: 57% of the erroneous classifications were in that category.

Table 9. Classification Table for Three Work-Setting Categories Based on MDF Analysis

Actual Group	Predicted Group		
	Solo	Group	Institutional
Solo	13 (36%)	7	16
Group	6	21 (45%)	20
Institutional	8	7	48 (76%)
Total	27	35	84

When the MDA was replicated for subsequent years in medical school, none of the analyses were significant. They did show the same pattern of being able to correctly identify about 80% of the physicians who chose to work in institutions but not being able to exceed chance on solo and group practitioners.

Summary and Conclusions

Solo practitioners were older when they started medical school, had lower GPAs and MCAT scores and were concrete thinkers who believed they should be more abstract. They were calm, easy-going individuals with practical goals and wanted to focus their efforts on direct patient care. Their academic performance was poorer than that of their peers. This group is similar to Quenk and Albert's "Traditional Primary Care Niche."

Solo Plus practitioners were serious and forthright but tense and easily upset. Their fathers were well-educated and they had more brothers than their average classmate. They wanted to spend less time in direct patient care and more on research. They were disinclined toward working in government institutions and not bothered by being far from a medical school. Their academic performance was slightly better than that of their peers.

Small Group practitioners tended to be warm, compassionate, trustworthy and liked to inspire others. They liked the idea of working on a joint project with other physicians and aspired to expand their medical knowledge. They believed that physicians should be more than an MD in their communities but their academic performance was poorer than that of their peers. This group was most similar to Quenk and Albert's "Physician Statesman Niche."

Medium-sized group practitioners were quiet, unassuming individuals who liked to focus on the practical needs of others and tended to be gentle in dealing with them. These no-nonsense practitioners did not want to learn about any of the "warm and fuzzy stuff" in regard to patients or in regard to themselves. They didn't want to be bothered with psycho-social matters in their practice or be otherwise involved in their community. They simply wanted to concentrate on what they considered their core task of helping patients in practical ways. Their academic performance was better than that of their peers

Large Group practitioners were self-disciplined, imaginative, tender-minded, compassionate, and inclined to strive for harmony in interpersonal relations. They were disinclined toward family practice and working with adults but liked the idea of teaching. They wanted more informal contact with faculty and more responsibility in directing their education. Although they had higher GPAs than their peers, their academic performance did not differ significantly

Hospital-based practitioners were cheerful and enthusiastic and liked novelty and the challenge of solving concrete biologic problems with unemotional logic. They were more group dependent that their peers, tending to be good followers. They were attracted to working with children but disinclined to teaching and solo private practice. Their academic performance was better than that of their peers.

University-based physicians knew they wanted to work in an educational environment from the start. They were serious, self-assured, restrained, and self-disciplined. They thought students should be enthusiastic about learning and show scholarship. They wanted to experience variety in their work tasks and achieved better academic performance than their peers. This group corresponds to Quenk and Albert's " Medical Teacher Niche."

Government practitioners were more likely to be introverted thinking types (logical, analytical, not swayed by emotional considerations). They had higher preferences for work in government hospitals and facilities and were disinclined toward large medical groups and teaching. They were not inclined toward academics or community participation and unconcerned about red tape, routine, or team work in their work setting. They wanted doctors to be respectful of patients and faculty to be respectful of them as students. Their academic performance was mixed. This group corresponds to the "Service-Institutional Niche" of Quenk and Albert.

Only students who eventually ended up practicing in institutions (hospitals, universities and government facilities) were able to accurately anticipate their work setting at the time they entered medical school. This is about 80% of 43% of the total students or about one third. On reflection, this perhaps should not be so surprising since medical students have not, for the most part, had direct experience of the features of group and solo practice and been able to evaluate their "fit" for themselves. These results and the more fine grained analysis using all eight categories indicates that work-setting selection is a much more fungible choice than that of medical specialty.

Gerald Otis and Naomi Quenk

5 THE WAY THEY WERE: PRACTICE COMMUNITIES

Gerald D. Otis

In 1996 Rivo and Kindig[62] noted there was a decrease in the number of primary care physicians in rural areas and the number of National Health Service Corps physicians who provided care to many of those under-served areas dropped from 2300 in 1979 to fewer than 200 in 1991. There were, in 2013, about 68 primary care physicians per 100,000 population in rural areas of the United States as opposed to about 84 in urban areas. The Robert Graham Center for Policy Studies in Family Medicine and Primary Care estimate that, in order to reach a standard of one primary care physician per 2000 citizens, an additional 2670 rural physicians are needed.

Back in 1970, Bible[63] noted that students from small towns were more likely to return to small towns to practice and Sax[64] reviewed the literature on programs intended to influence that choice. Rabinowitz[65] noted that taking a rural clinical rotation during medical school was the strongest predictor of a subsequent decision to practice in a rural community. I did a path analysis of the effects of MECO preceptorships on medical student dispositions toward small town practice[66] and found that size of town of origin, size of preceptorship community, and initial dispositions all affected post preceptorship dispositions toward small town practice but that size of community of origin had the greatest cumulative effect due to its indirect effects on the other variables. Similar findings were obtained in Australia[67].

Elam et al.[68] found that a significant percentage of their students returned to practice in the district where they grew up in Kentucky while Looney et al.[69], in the same state, found they could predict who would *not* choose a rural area but not those who would.

Perhaps the most detailed investigation of rural practitioners has been done by Bowman [70, 71, 72, 73, 74]. He found that *students* interested in rural practice not only were more likely to have grown up in rural areas but were older, married, white, more likely to choose rotations away from major medical centers, and did volunteer work twice as often as other students. He believed these students were stable, mature and service oriented. Rural *physicians* were more likely to be male, white or Native, older, rural born, family practitioners who attended osteopathic or public medical schools. Forty-three percent of rural born family practitioners practice in a rural location and those who went to a family practice residency program with a rural training emphasis were even more likely to practice in a rural location. Bowman noted that, working against recruiting more physicians for rural practice is the fact that currently less than 10% of student admissions are rural born. And medical schools that focus on academics, youth, research, serving the elite, and that do not have a rural mission or a family practice program with rural placements during training do nothing to stem the tide away from rural practice.

The American Association of Family Practice[75] has proposed that medical schools increase recruitment of students from rural settings, teach survival skills for practicing in rural communities, include rural components in medical training and offer a rural training track in graduate medical education, and seek funding for rural medical education from all sources. They point out that the increase in the number of women in medical schools, who usually do not select rural practice, may require some adjustments. They also note that those who feel better prepared for rural practice, both medically (e. g., for lack of support services) and socially (especially for the lack of anonymity) are twice as likely to remain for at least six years. Education with respect to the business aspects of medical practice in rural areas and the resources available are also seen as desirable.

The present study investigates the associations between chosen size of practice community of a group of end-of-career physicians and many features of these same physicians at the time they entered medical school nearly half a century earlier.

Methods

Subjects, data, and analytical procedures (salience analysis, treatment of MBTI data, and multiple discriminant function analysis) are all the same as those described in the previous two chapters.

The population size for each community was looked up on Wikipedia. The size of the communities in which doctors practiced was divided into four categories: less than 50,000 population (27%); from 50,000 to 120,000 population (16%); 120,000 to 500,000 population (19%); and over 500,000 population (39%). Suburban areas that were part of a larger metropolitan area were placed in the largest population category (> 500K). Thus, a little over a quarter of graduates chose to practice in small towns (< 50K) but over a third chose to practice in a large metropolitan area or a suburb of one.

Results of Salience Analysis for Selection of Practice Community

Small Towns Practice (population of 50,000 or less)

Medical students who would subsequently choose to practice in towns under 50,000 population were more likely to have already decided upon the type of work they wanted to do (presumably clinical) at the time they began their career (.00), with the proviso that they be able to control their patient load (.01). They were less inclined to select Cardiology (.04) or Surgery (.00) as a specialty, were disinclined to work in a government facility (.01) but practice in an industrial setting (.04) or in a foreign country (.04) appealed to them. Three of their ratings are somewhat puzzling: they were less inclined than their peers to want to work with adolescents (.03), adults (.01) or all ages of patients unselectively (.02). They thought the geographic location of their practice community (.01) and its distance from a large metropolitan area was important (.02) in their decision-making. They rated population size as important in selecting a practice community (.02) and were disinclined to practice in a large metropolitan area (.04). It was not important to them how far from a medical school they were (.02) and they were disinclined to practice in a community with a fast pace of life (.04). They were drawn to work in a community with a moderate average income (.00). As students, these practitioners spent more of their leisure time recreating with family members only (.01) or engaged in meetings of civic, church, political or other task-oriented groups (.03).

Small town practitioners had lower scores on the MCAT General Information Scale (.04). Nineteen percent of small town practitioners were from communities with a population of 25,000 or less while 40% were from a large city. (Looked at from the other direction, 30% of subjects from a town of 25,000 or less ended up practicing in a town of 50,000 or less vs 22% of subjects from a large city who did so). This is the same relationship found in earlier studies.

Small town practitioners were more likely to be classified as the ESFP Psychological Type on the MBTI (.000) and less likely to be classified as INFP (.015). ESFPs are said to be "exuberant lovers of life." They are practical, realistic and tactful. They are good team players and often peace-makers. They are not fond of theories and traditional schools may be difficult for them. They were less likely to have the IP two-point code (.022) and the I_FP three-point code (.017). They were more likely to have the EP two-point code (.009) and to have the ES_P three-point code (.022) on the MBTI.

On the SFRQ, small town practitioners tended to score higher on the Recognition Scale (importance of students receiving recognition for their accomplishments, that their individuality be recognized, that they are understood and appreciated as individuals) (.05). They had significantly higher scores on the PIQ Community Orientation Scale (the degree to which the respondent considers it important that the physician be involved in health-related community activities other than patient care) (.02).

Performances on academic measures were lower for this group. They had lower ratings by faculty in their clerkship rotations for Surgery(.01), Pediatrics (.01) and Psychiatry (.03). They scored lower on National Boards, Part 1, Biology (.04), Microbiology (.01) and Pharmacology (.00) sections. On Part 2 of National Boards they scored lower on the Surgery (.03), Pediatrics (.05) and Physical Medicine (.01) sections.

Medium Town Practice 1 (50,000 to 120,000 population)

Physicians who chose to practice in towns between 50,000 and 120,000 population, as entering medical students, preferred to practice in the Rocky Mountain region (.01) and were inclined toward large group practice (.01). They were disinclined toward working in a military setting (.04). It was not important for them to be near prominent persons in their field of medicine (.04) and the prestige of their medical organization was also not important to them (.02). As students, they spent less of their leisure time on informal outings with friends than did their peers (.00).

Medium-sized town selectors were more likely to have had a college major in one of the biological sciences (.01). The educational attainment of both parents was lower (.01, .00) and their fathers were less likely to be physicians (.02).

These respondents did not distinguish themselves on the MCAT or with respect to GPAs. They scored lower on the 16PF Guilt Proneness Scale (more self-assured, less self-reproaching) (.00) and the Tender-mindedness Scale (more tough-minded, self-reliant, no-nonsense, less sensitive) (.01).

They scored lower on four of the SFRQ Scales: Structure (importance of faculty giving prompt feedback, specifying what is required, encouraging questions, giving recognition, evaluating by means of regular tests) (.00), Faculty Socio-emotional Role (the degree to which faculty should go out of their way to be helpful to students, be friendly and supportive, help them to work out problems and understand themselves, etc.) (.05), Faculty Respectfulness (being considerate of patients during interviews and examinations, requesting their permission for procedures to be carried out, explaining procedures; also, the importance of faculty being "good examples" in their dealings with patients, being patient with students who don't understand, respecting individual student interests, etc.) (.05), and Faculty Teacher Efficiency (the importance of faculty exciting student curiosity through teaching, specifying course requirements, accommodating to student needs, encouraging questions and discussion, giving prompt feedback, having courses well organized, being good speakers, etc.) (.00). Their scores on all of these scales is consistent with their no-nonsense, tough-minded, self-reliant disposition evident on the 16PF: no coddling of students required! On the PIQ they were disinclined toward coddling patients either: they were more likely to have higher scores than their peers on the Disease Orientation Scale (importance for the physician to focus his efforts on the treatment of biological disease rather than becoming involved in preventive and psycho-social medicine) (.01).

Doctors who chose to practice in communities of this size were rated lower on Clinical Science during their second year (.03) but had higher scores on National Boards, Part 1, Biology (.05). Otherwise, they did not distinguish themselves on the performance measures.

Medium Town Practice 2 (120,000 to 500,000 population)

When looking forward to their future careers, students who eventually decided to practice in communities with populations of from 120,000 to 500,000 were less inclined to select Family Medicine (.03) or OBGYN (.04) as specialties, to work in an educational setting (.03) or to work with the geriatric population (.01). They did not consider the size of the community an important factor in making their career decisions (.01) but did consider the frequency of the need to meet emergencies to be so (.00). They were more disposed than their peers toward practicing in a suburb (.01) and being in a high demand/low supply area for their specialty (.01).

Selectors of this size community were less likely to have majored in a biological science in college (.02) and less likely to have had any work experience in a medical setting (.02). Their fathers were less likely to have been a physician (.03) and neither parent was likely to have worked in a medical field (.02). Their families of origin contained more girls than the families of their peers (.01).

These respondents tended to have higher scores on the MCAT Quantitative Scale (.00). Their scores on the 16PF Control Scale were higher (more socially precise, self-disciplined, compulsive) (.05) as were their scores on the IQ Scale (more abstract, less concrete thinkers) (.05). They scored lower on the 16PF Happy-go-lucky Scale (more enthusiastic, less serious or prudent) (.03). On the MBTI they scored higher on the EI Scale (more Introverted, reflective, focus in depth vs broadly, private and contained) (.04) and lower on the TF Scale (more Thinking, logical, analytical, fairness oriented) (.03).

Choosers of this size community did not distinguish themselves on any of the SFRQ Scales. On the Physician Ideology Questionnaire they scored lower than their classmates on Psychosocial Orientation (importance for the physician to have knowledge and skill in interpersonal relations and apply that knowledge and skill to the social and emotional problems of patients) (.05), lower on Biological Orientation (importance attached to the physician's biological knowledge and skill in applying it) (.02) and higher on the Disease Orientation Scale (importance for the physician to focus his efforts on the treatment of biological disease rather than becoming involved in preventive and psycho-social medicine) (.04).

The only distinguishing feature these respondents had on the performance measures was that they had higher clerkship ratings for their Psychiatry rotation (.01).

Large City Practitioners (500,000 + population)

Physicians who ended up practicing in a large city, as entering medical students, showed their preference for big city living: they rated distance from a large metropolitan area as more important to them than did their peers in deciding upon a practice community (.02) and gave higher ratings to their preference for practicing in such a community (.04). Pace of life was important to them in selecting a practice community (.05). Although they considered community economic status as less important (.04), they preferred to live in a community with a moderate average income (.00). They showed a lesser preference for living on the West Coast than other students (.03).

Large city practitioners were more inclined toward the basic sciences (.00), OBGYN (.03) and Pediatrics (.05). They had a greater inclination to work with children (.01) and neonates (.02) and considered the type of patients they would be working with as more important than did their classmates (.02). They considered the ability to control patient load (.03) and working hours (.02) as less important as was being in a high demand/low supply area for their particular specialty (.01). Big city doctors, as students, were less inclined to work in a foreign country (.01) and more inclined to work in a government facility (.03) or government health program (.01), although work in a non-government facility was also acceptable to them (.02).

Physicians who chose to work in a large city were more likely to be female (.05) and had parents who were both more likely to be employed in a health profession (.01). Their fathers' educational attainment was likely to be higher than that of their peers (.00). There tended to be fewer siblings in their families of origin (.04). These respondents scored higher on the MCAT General Information (.01) and Quantitative (.03) Scales than did samples of randomly selected medical students. Fifty-one percent of large city practitioners were from large cities while 13% were from small towns. (Looked at from the opposite angle, 46% of students who grew up in a large city returned to a large city to practice medicine while 22% ended up practicing in a small town).

On the 16PF, students who eventually practiced in large cities scored lower on the Control Scale (less self-disciplined more careless of protocol, more inclined to follow their own urges) (.03). They scored higher on the Outgoing Scale (easy-going, warmhearted, more inclined to participate) (.00) and the Tender-mindedness Scale (less self-reliant, less realistic, more sensitive and dependent) (.00). They also achieved higher scores on the MBTI TF Scale (more toward the Feeling end of the scale: empathic, compassionate, warm-hearted) (.05).

Big city doctors, as entering medical students, had higher scores on the SFRQ Psychosocial Orientation Scale (importance of learning about psychological, social, and cultural factors in so far as they are relevant to patient care and augment clinical ability) (.05) and they also had higher scores on the PIQ Psychosocial Orientation Scale (importance of the physician having knowledge and skill in interpersonal relations and applying that knowledge and skill to the social and emotional problems of patients) (.02). They also scored higher on the PIQ Community Orientation Scale (physician should be involved in health-related community activities other than patient care) (.04).

Students who ended up practicing in large cities had higher Success Indexes for year 1 (.03) and higher ratings for their performance in their clerkship rotations in Medicine (.00), Pediatrics (.01) and OBGYN (.01). On National Boards, Part 1, they had higher scores than their peers in Pathology (.04), Microbiology (.00) and Pharmacology (.00) while on Part 2 of the National Boards they scored higher on the Medicine (.01), Pediatrics (.03), Physical Medicine (.05) and Psychiatry (.05) sections.

Multiple Discriminant Function Analysis for Choice of Practice Community

One-way analyses of variance for seven of the career preference variables used in the MDA showed a significant difference between the community categories: importance of size in selecting a practice community (p = .016), importance of pace of life (p = .013), being in a high demand/low supply area (p = .008), being near prominent people in your field of medicine (p = .003), the kind of patients to be served (p = .005), frequency of need to meet emergencies (p = .050), and opportunity to practice in a foreign country (p = .007). Results of the MDA for selection of practice community size appears in Table 10.

Table 10. Results of MDA Analysis for Choice of Size of Practice Community

No.	Root	Proportion	Canonical R	Chi-Squared	D.F.	Probabilities
1	0.5967	0.5858	0.6113	132.6420	45	0.000
2	0.2792	0.2741	0.4672	59.4118	28	0.000
3	0.1427	0.1401	0.3534	20.8816	13	0.075

As can be seen, the analysis produced two significant discriminant functions along with one that was just shy of significance. The canonical correlation of 0.6113 represents a substantial degree of association between the linear combination of predictor variables and the practice community size array variable.

Cross tabulation between predicted category assignment and observed category membership is shown in Table 11. The table shows that the best prediction was for the most populous category, Large City, with 86% accuracy. (If you bet that everyone would end up in a big city, you would be right only 51% of the time). The next best prediction was for towns with from 120,000 to 500,000 citizens. Predictions for small town practice logged in at 56% while the poorest prediction rate was for towns from 50,000 to 120,000 in population (32%). The discriminant functions were biased toward over-predicting members in the Large City category and under-predicting membership in small towns and towns between 50,000 and 120,000 citizens. Overall, the percent of correct placements for practice community size was an impressive 69%. Thus, it looks like most medical students, when just beginning their career, had a very good idea of the size of the community in which they would eventually practice.

Table 11. Classification Table for Predicted and Actual Community Size Groups

Actual Group	Predicted Group			
	Small Town	Med Comm1	Med Comm2	Large City
Small Town	20 (56%)	1	2	13
Med Comm1	2	7 (32%)	3	10
Med Comm2	3	0	15 (63%)	6
Large City	5	4	3	73 (86%)
Total	30 (18%)	12 (7%)	23 (14%)	102 (61%)

Again, one might expect there to be an association between size of chosen practice community and specialty, but that does not appear to be the case except for one combination of community size and specialty cluster (see Table 12). The chi-square value for the table as a whole is not significant but individuals who chose specialties falling into the Technique and Instrument Cluster chose to live in communities between 50,000 and 120,000 twice as often as expected (p = 0.01).

Table 12. Cross tabulation between community size and specialty cluster.

Specialty Cluster	Small Town	Med Comm1	Med Comm2	Large City	Total
Internal Medicine	14 (16.9)	12 (9.6)	11 (9.0)	26 (27.5)	63 (19%)
Surgery	9 (7.8)	1 (4.4)	6 (4.2)	13 (12.6)	29 (9%)
Family Medicine	31 (27.9)	13 (15.8)	14 (14.9)	46 (45.3)	104 (31%)

Tech. & Inst.	10 (11.3)	13 (6.4)	3 (6.0)	16 (18.3)	42 (13%)
Psychiatry	4 (9.4)	6 (5.3)	6 (5.0)	19 (15.3)	35 (10%)
Diagnostic	14 (10.7)	3 (6.1)	6 (5.7)	17 (17.4)	40 (12%)
OBGYN	8 (5.9)	3 (3.3)	2 (3.2)	9 (9.6)	22 (7%)
Total	90 (27%)	51 (15%)	48 (14%)	146 (44%)	335

Note: except for the bottom row and rightmost column, numbers in parentheses are expected values.

Finally, one may wonder if there is a relationship between work-setting choices and practice community size choices. The cross-tabulation between these variables is given in Table 13. The overall chi square (for the whole table) with 21 degrees of freedom was significant at the .002 level indicating a small but highly significant association between practice type and size of practice community. The contingency coefficient was 0.345 and Cramer's V was 0.212. University-based practices were over-represented by nearly twice the number expected in large cities and were under-represented in small towns by a factor of 11, as one might expect. Just barely short of significance was the association between small town and solo private practice (the chi square was 3.807 while a value of 3.841 was required for significance at the .05 level). Also just shy of significance was the association between towns of 50,000 to 120,000 and solo private practice with hospital associations and university-based practices.

Table 13. Cross tabulation between community size and practice type (work-setting).

Practice Type	Small Town	Med Comm1	Med Comm2	Large City	Totall
Solo	25 (17) †	7 (9.8)	10 (8.9)	22 (28.3)	64
Solo+	5 (8.2)	9 (4.8) †	5 (4.3)	12 (13.7)	31
Small Group	16 (13.5)	7 (7.8)	7 (7.1)	21 (22.6)	51
Medium Group	5 (6.6)	6 (3.8)	2 (3.5)	12 (11.1)	25
Large Group	2 (2.7)	2 (1.5)	1 (1.4)	5 (4.4)	10
Hospital-based	25 (21.5)	15 (12.4)	11 (11.2)	30 (35.9)	81
University-based	1 (11.4) **	2 (6.6) †	5 (6)	35 (19) ***	43
Government	9 (7.2)	3 (4.1)	5 (3.7)	10 (12)	27
Total	88	51	46	147	332

† Significant between .10 and .05 level. ** Significant at .005 level. *** Significant at .001 level

Summary and Conclusions

Results of the study indicated that, although most small town practitioners grew up in a larger town, those from a small town had a greater probability of ending up in a small town to practice. They are practical and realistic individuals who are team players and often tactful peace-makers. As students, they disliked surgery or cardiology as specialty choices, disliked government employment or living in a large community but were community-oriented and wanted to receive recognition for their accomplishments. Geographic location, population size and distance from a medical school were important factors in their career decision-making. Their academic performance was poorer than that of their peers.

Physicians who chose to practice in communities between 50K and 120K in population were of a no-nonsense, tough-minded, self-reliant disposition and, consistent with that, they didn't think students required any coddling. They were disinclined toward coddling patients either, believing it important for the physician to focus his efforts on the treatment of biological disease rather than becoming involved in preventive and psycho-social medicine. They were likely to have majored in a biological science as an undergraduate and were unconcerned about the prestige of their medical organization or being near prominent people in their field of medicine. They wanted to stay in the Rocky Mountain Region and preferred large group practice. Their performance on academic measures was not remarkable.

Physicians who chose to practice in communities between 120K and 500K in population were disinclined toward family medicine or obstetrics as specialties, work in an educational setting or with geriatric patients but they preferred practicing in a suburb. They did not consider size of community to be important but thought the frequency of need to meet emergencies was a consideration in choosing a practice site. Self-disciplined and enthusiastic, they were likely to be reflective, logical and analytical abstract thinkers. They were less likely to have majored in a biological science and were from a family with a greater number of girls than their peers but one whose parents were not employed in a medical field. They were neither biologically nor psycho-socially oriented but believed the physician should concentrate his efforts on treating disease.

Physicians who chose to work in a large city were more likely to be female with fewer siblings and had parents who were both more likely to be employed in a health profession. They had higher scores on two MCAT scales and were inclined toward basic medical science, obstetrics, pediatrics, working with children, living in a big city and government employment. They were not concerned about controlling patient load or hours but pace of life and distance from a metropolitan area were important considerations for them. They tended to be less self-disciplined, more easy-going, warmhearted, sensitive and empathic than their peers. They showed better academic performance on many measures than did their classmates.

Results of the multiple discriminate analysis on selection of size of community in which to practice produced two significant discriminant functions and an overall concordance rate of 69%. Best prediction was for practice in a large city (86%) and poorest was for practice in a community of between 50,000 and 120,000 population (32%). Fifty-six percent of the small town practitioners were predictable from their entry level ratings of 15 practice community characteristics. Thus, the majority of students know the size of the communities that will eventually become their practice communities at the time they enter medical school.

6 SOURCES OF PHYSICIAN SATISFACTION BY SPECIALTY

Naomi Quenk, Ph.D.

Current national concern with increasing the availability of medical care has generally concentrated on such potential solutions as the recruitment of medical students from minority groups, providing financial incentives for practice in under-served areas, utilization of physician extenders in areas with few-physicians, and the like. Though general knowledge is available concerning the negative qualities of certain practice settings, such as the lack of adequate referral facilities in remote rural areas, life style deficiencies in inner city areas, and low salaries in certain institutional settings, little is known about the specific characteristics of differing physician work settings which are associated with satisfaction and dissatisfaction. As a result, any attempts to modify the opportunities in existing settings, or create innovative forms of health care delivery, must be based upon the available fund of general knowledge or on assumptions which have not yet been proven valid.

The present study is an attempt to provide in a detailed fashion, a description of the kinds of activities and characteristics which are associated with physician satisfaction and dissatisfaction. Such knowledge can permit a better understanding of physician motivation and may serve as a useful guide to increasing the potential for satisfaction in a variety of physician work situations.

Data for the study were available in the form of responses to the Physician Work Setting Instrument (PWSI), a questionnaire designed to assess the frequency of medical activities as well as the extent to which, in addition, the physician revealed his satisfaction with each item by indicating whether he would like it to be more frequent or characteristic, less frequent or characteristic, the same, or whether it was irrelevant. The sum of the items the physician indicated he would like to remain the same was used as a measure of overall satisfaction in the present study.

Method

Sample

The 477 physician respondents to the Physician Work Setting Study (Quenk and Albert, 1975)[76] , constituted the sample for this study. These physicians had been selected to represent 14 medical specialties including general and family practice; 11 practice organizations, including various forms of private practice and several institutional settings; 5 community sizes; and 5 states representing the five geographic regions of the United States.

The response rate for this sample was approximately 40% of those sampled. Analysis of non-responders to the study indicated no significant differences for the variables available for comparison. These were: age, year of graduation from medical school, medical school attended, board certification, membership in specialty societies, community size, type of practice and practice organization.

Data Analysis Techniques

For the purpose of developing the Taxonomy of Physician Work Settings, rating of the frequency and characteristicness of the 62 items of the PWSI were cluster analyzed using the BC-TRY system of cluster analysis (Tryon and Bailey, 1970)[77]. This method resulted in 7 distinct clusters each of which scores on these clusters were used as variables in the present study. Table 14 presents in detail the clusters and the items contained in each.

Table 14. PWSI - Activities and Characteristics of Work Settings

Cluster I - **"Personal Patient Involvement"** (Reliability = .8730)	
Item	Factor Coefficient
*Advising or counseling patients and/or their families	0.8660
*Direct patient contact	0.7951
*Dealing with patients' emotional difficulties	0.7387
*Explaining diagnoses and treatment plans to patients and their families	0.6942
*Opportunity to follow and evaluate patient progress	0.6616
Referring patients to other practitioners or institutions	0.6054
Performing therapeutic procedures including surgery, psychotherapy, radiologic treatment, etc.	0.4907
Maintaining a fairly consistent and predictable patient scheduling system	0.4562
Opportunity for appreciation and prestige from the lay public	0.4140
Emphasis on diagnosing and developing treatment plans	0.4085
Devoting time to particular patient problems or kinds of patients	0.3818
Medical record keeping	0.3644
Cluster 2 - "Physician-Teacher" (Reliability= .8273)	

Item	Factor Coefficient
*Teaching medical students, interns or residents	0.8243
*Supervision and/or teaching medical students or medical personnel (e.g., paramedics)	0.7375
*Opportunity for affiliation with a medical school	0.7013
*Presenting cases to some audience	0.6297
Organizational administration (e. g., committee work, policy development)	0.4412
Supervision of subordinates	0.4222

Cluster 3 - "Personal Control of Professional Situation" (Reliability= .7937)

Items	Factor Coefficient
*Maintaining my preferred "pace of life"	0.8092
*Sufficient time for family and/or outside activities	0.8004
*Determining amount of free time and/or vacation time	0.7076
*Cultural or recreational activities in my geographical area	0.4020

Cluster 4 - "Medical Innovation" (Reliability= .7522)

Items	Factor Coefficient
*Trying out new ideas	0.7279
*Access to new developments in a field of interest or specialization	0.6594
*Expanding one's own knowledge in an area of medicine	0.6240
*Dealing with new or unusual patient problems	0.5596
Delegation of certain medical tasks to subordinates	0.3796

Cluster 5 - "Personal Control of Income" (Reliability= .6667)

Items	Factor Coefficient
*Personally handling financial aspects of medical practice	0.7071
*Personal control of amount of earnings	0.7052
Personal control of amount of time devoted to patient care	0.3503

Cluster 6 - "Interaction with the Medical Community" (Reliability .6992)

Items	Factor Coefficient
*Working with other physicians on some joint task	0.0688
*Sharing patient responsibility with other physicians	0.6435
*Dealing with emergency medical problems	0.4851
*Sharing doubts, frustrations or problems with colleagues	0.4586
*Access to hospital facilities	0.4004
Accessibility of consultation services	0.4172

Cluster 7 - "Professional Ambition" (Reliability= .7420)

Items	Factor Coefficient
*Opportunity for professional advancement	0.7866
*Focus on a special interest area within a specialty	0.5917
*Opportunity for prestige and recognition from colleagues	0.5816
*Intellectual stimulation through interaction with colleagues	0.5332

*items are definers of the clusters. Cluster scores are based on definers only.

Data were analyzed in several ways in order to provide both general information as well as detailed descriptions of sources of satisfaction and dissatisfaction for physicians in general as well as specific subgroups (e. g, medical specialties and practice organizations).

For analyses that required creation of a satisfied group for comparison with a dissatisfied group the following criteria were used: for the total sample. the satisfied group required an individual satisfaction score ½ standard deviation above the mean for the sample; a dissatisfied physician had a score ½ standard deviation below the mean for the sample. For all other subgroups, the satisfied group had a score above the mean and the dissatisfied group a score below the mean. This less extreme breakdown was necessary for subgroups in order to maintain sufficient sample members for adequate analysis.

Three statistical techniques were used, although not all groupings received all three forms of treatment:

- Discriminant function analysis, which was performed only for total sample satisfaction. This technique identified those variables which maximally differentiated between the satisfied and dissatisfied groups of physicians.
- Multiple regression analysis, which identified the set of variables which maximally correlated with the criterion of satisfaction. This was performed for total sample, specialties and some practice organizations.

- The t-test which identified those variables which significantly differentiated between satisfied and dissatisfied physicians. This technique was used for all groups.

Results

Total Sample

The total samples of satisfied and dissatisfied physicians were compared using the t-.test on all clusters as well as on all individual items not appearing in any cluster. In addition, community size variables, length of time in setting, patient load, income, age and year of graduation from medical school were included as potential variables which might be associated with satisfaction. The sum of items rated irrelevant, less characteristic and more characteristic were included as an index of the extent and nature of dissatisfaction.

Table 15 indicates that the satisfied physicians were raised in larger communities, earn more money, are younger, and have higher scores on all clusters except Personal Patient Involvement. Examination of specific items which significantly discriminated the two groups leads to the observation that satisfied physicians have a greater degree of control over their working and personal lives, better communication within the medical community, in the form of available consultation and interaction with other professionals, and have a greater amount of independence in their work situations.

The variables selected for inclusion in this and subsequent analyses of satisfied versus dissatisfied physicians focus on both general and detailed aspects of practice characteristics, including specific items as well as clusters. Variables such as age were included in order to observe whether era effects may be influencing any differences in practice characteristics. Myers-Briggs Type Indicator variables were also included as potential discriminators, particularly for specialty subgroups. Because regression analysis with small samples cannot validly handle large numbers of variables, the equations are based upon a more limited set of descriptors.

Thus Table 16 (and regression tables for all subgroups) included the seven clusters, income, community size, length of time in setting and patient load as important descriptors of practice setting, and Myers-Briggs Type Indicator continuous scores, pre-college community size and year of graduation from medical school as important personality and background characteristics. In order to permit ease of comparison across the various groups studied, the same set of variables was entered for all regression analyses.

Table 15. Means, Standard Deviations and significance levels for satisfied (N=123) versus Dissatisfied (N=150) Physicians

	Satisfied		Dissatisfied			
Variable	Mean	SD	Mean	SD	t	p
Pre-college Community Size	2.99	1.54	2.49	1.48	2.71	<.005
Community size	4.00	1.13	3.87	1.20	0.89	ns
Time in present setting	8.23	6.13	8.07	6.61	0.20	ns

Income	4.14	1.02	3.87	1.15	1.92	<.05
Number of patients seen per week	104.84	85.33	108.31	87.91	0.31	ns
Age of Physician	43.30	6.12	44.85	6.79	1.82	<.05
Year graduation from medical school	55.94	7.64	54.97	8.76	0.97	ns
Personal Patient Involvement	51.29	9.40	49.27	10.93	1.62	ns
Physician Teacher	51.18	10.40	47.29	11.54	2.90	<.005
Personal Control of Professional Situation	52.95	10.18	44.59	14.76	5.35	<.005
Medical Innovation	52.42	9.57	46.10	14.88	4.09	<.005
Personal Control of Income	51.93	10.40	47.30	14.06	3.04	<.005
Interaction with the medical community	52.63	9.63	45.76	14.41	4.54	<.005
Professional Prestige	52.40	9.72	44.93	14.23	4.97	<.005
Keeping a fairly consistent and predictable scheduling system	4.97	1.32	4.16	1.75	4.05	<.005
Working alone (little assistance from other medical personnel)	2.33	1.73	3.29	1.91	4.27	<.005
Performing therapeutic procedures	3.39	1.73	3.75	1.66	1.73	<.05
Devoting time to particular patient problems or kinds of patients	4.36	1.54	4.01	1.68	1.78	<.05
Satisfactory coverage during periods of absence	5.51	1.11	4.83	1.60	3.98	<.005
Responsibility for defining one's role, duties and activities	5.08	1.21	4.46	1.56	3.54	<.005
Dealing with patient's emotional difficulties	4.25	1.64	4.01	1.77	1.13	ns
Opportunity for appreciation and prestige from the lay public	4.14	1.66	3.67	1.75	2.27	<.025
Availability of consultation services	5.66	0.81	5.08	1.25	4.39	<.005
Isolation from other physicians	1.47	1.15	2.35	1.68	4.83	<.005
Time "wasted" due to travel between professional locations	2.13	1.52	2.63	1.86	2.39	<.025
Taking less vacation and/or free time than one is entitled to take	2.91	1.75	3.48	1.91	2.50	<.025

Variable					
Availability of desirable public school system	5.05	1.30	4.32	1.67	3.88	<.005
Opportunities for spouse to be employed or pursue preferred activities	4.85	1.52	3.84	1.88	4.65	<.005
Active participation in non-medical community affairs	3.9	1.6	3.4	1.76	2.4	<.025
Opportunity to follow and evaluate patient progress	5.25	1.22	4.81	1.40	2.72	<.005

The regression technique proceeds by initially selecting the variable which by itself accounts for the largest amount of the variance contained in the data. It then continues to add additional variables on the basis of the amount of variance each contributes, while taking into account the correlation of that variable with those already considered. The result after all variables have been included is the total amount of variance explained by the variables included in the equation. Variables which are found to contribute less than a predetermined amount to the equation are not included. For that reason, the various equations to be reported vary in the number of elements in the equation.

The Beta Weights reported indicate the importance of each variable in relation to the criterion of satisfaction. They are reported in ascending order such that the first listed is the most important to the equation. The total variance reported at the bottom of the table is not based upon the Beta Weights but reflects how much of the available variation is explained by the total set of variables in the equation.

In Table 16, the most important contributor to overall satisfaction is cluster 3 - "Personal Control of the Professional Situation." However. only 16% of the total variance is explained using the 15 variables in the equation.

Table 16. Regression Equation Predicting Satisfaction for the Total Sample of Physicians (N•477)

Variable	Beta Wt.
Cluster 3 - Personal control of professional situation	0.2339
Cluster 6 - Interaction with medical community	0.0991
Thinking-Feeling (Feeling direction)	0.0965
Cluster 2- Physician - Teacher	0.0857
Pre-college community size (larger communities)	0.0773
Average number patients seen per week	-0.0669
Cluster 7 - Professional prestige	0.0631
Income	0.0619
Judgment - Perception (judgmental direction)	-0.5292

Cluster 5 - Personal control of income	0.0500
Year of graduation from medical school	0.0487
Extraversion - Introversion (Extraverted direction)	-0.0248
Sensing • Intuition (Intuitive direction	0.0234
Cluster 1 - Personal patient involvement	0.0120
Community size (smaller communities)	-0.0076
TOTAL VARIANCE	0.1607

(A negative beta weight indicates that a low score on the variable is correlated with satisfaction).

Thus, the ability of this technique to adequately explain overall satisfaction for the total sample is poor. As will be seen, predictive ability improves considerably in analyses of subgroups, primarily due to increased variability among sub-group members. For the total sample, which includes all specialties, all practice organizations and all personality types, the particular variables selected for inclusion in the regression equation are inadequate to predict satisfaction.

A third method of examining satisfaction was the discriminant function analysis. This procedure, based (as were the t-tests) on the two groups of satisfied and dissatisfied physicians, identifies those variables which maximally discriminate between the two groups. In essence, the method selects those variables on which the groups are " farthest apart", and stops considering variables when the extent of separation becomes insignificant. Table 17 reports the discriminate function coefficients of the variables found to discriminate the two groups, in descending order of importance.

Table 17. Standardized Discriminant Function Coefficients for Variables Maximally discriminating Satisfied from Dissatisfied Physicians (Total Sample)

Variable	Coefficient
Isolation from other physicians (item)	-0.5312
Cluster 3 - Personal control of professional situation	0.5045
Working alone (item)	-0.4341
Pre-college community size	0.3883
Serious financial constraints limiting provision of patient care (item)	-0.3658
Average number of patients seen per week	-0.2572
Availability of desirable public school system	0.2384
Cluster 4- Medical innovation	0.2187

Opportun1ty for spouse to be employed or pursue preferred activities	0.2013
Responsibility for defining one's role, duties and activities (item)	0.1432
Devoting time to particular patient problems or kinds of' patients (item)	0.1426

It should be noted that in this analysis, personality variables were not included, the focus being on practice characteristics. As in the previous two analyses, it appears that the variables which best discriminate the groups deal with the extent to which physicians feel isolated from the larger medical community and their (probably related) ability to control their work situation and personal lives. Thus the three analyses, though differing somewhat in the amount of detail provided, present a consistent picture of the satisfiers and dissatisfiers of physicians in general.

Tables 18 through 43 provide t-test results comparing the satisfied versus the dissatisfied groups within each of the specialties included in the sample, as well as regression equations predicting satisfaction for each specialty. In attempting to interpret these tables, a few comments are necessary.

In interpreting Myers-Briggs variables which appear, it is important to bear in mind that in the t-tests reported, raw scores indicating amount of each preference are used, as well as the continuous scores which show the strength of each preference in a particular direction. Thus, if one group is reported as being higher in extraversion, it does not mean that there are necessarily more extraverted types in the group, but rather that the mean extraversion score for the group is higher. For the regression equations, only the continuous score for each pair of preferences was included. Therefore, the direction noted where type preference appears in an equation indicates that the indicated direction is associated with satisfaction-for the group.

Second, unlike the t-tests for the total sample where only those items which did not appear in clusters were used for analysis, the analyses of subgroups included all available items in order to better describe differences in detailed fashion. Thus, where a particular cluster ,has been found to significantly differentiate the group, it is usually the case that al1 or most items in the cluster also appear in the t-test table.(Note: No analyses were performed with the group of 19 neurosurgeons as the sample available was too small for meaningful statistical treatment. Because of the way the Type Indicator is scored, there is not a perfect negative correlation between each pair of preferences. Therefore, it is possible for significance to occur for only one of a preference pair).

The procedure in describing the results of analyses for the specialties will be to note those variables which appear to be most important in relation to satisfaction, and where appropriate to discuss comparisons with other specialties in terms of interesting similarities or differences.

Specialties

Pediatricians (Tables 18 and 19)

In examining levels of significance for items discriminating the satisfied and dissatisfied groups, it is notable that only one achieves significance at less than the .01 level. Thus, differences between the two groups are not extreme and we might conclude that the two groups are not markedly dissimilar. However, satisfied pediatricians have been in their present setting a shorter time, work more often with other physicians and have greater opportunity to gain recognition from their colleagues. Although the two groups do not differ significantly on any of the seven clusters, in the regression equation· predicting satisfaction, "Personal Control of the Professional Situation" is most important while seeing fewer patients is second. As will be seen, one or both of these variables appears to be of leading importance particularly for specialties that are typically characterized by large patient loads.

Table 18. Pediatricians N=42 (S=21; D=21)

Variable	Satisfied		Dissatisfied			
	Mean	SD	Mean	SD	t	p
Time in present setting	4.81	2.96	7.65	6.60	1.79	<.10
Items rated irrelevant	2.05	2.01	4.68	6.00	1.90	<.10
Items Dr. wants "less characteristic"	5.80	3.04	7.95	4.76	1.70	<.10
Items Dr. wants "more characteristic"	13.48	5.22	30.14	9.43	7.08	<.01
Works alone	2.62	1.66	3.86	2.03	2.16	<.05
Performing diagnostic procedures	3.81	1.44	2.63	1.83	2.35	<.05
Presenting cases to some audience	3.24	1.34	2.45	1.28	1.92	<.10
Financial constraints limiting provision of patient care	2.57	1.60	3.01	1.70	2.62	<.05
Sharing patient responsibility with other physicians	5.14	0.85	4.33	1.35	2.32	<.05
Opportunity for prestige and recognition from colleagues	4.52	1.12	3.53	1.65	2.26	<.05
Working with or under a community board or citizen group	2.24	1.58	3.29	1.85	1.98	<.10
Cultural or recreational activities in my geographical area	5.10	0.79	4.38	1.60	1.81	<.10

Table 19. - Regression Equation Predicting Satisfaction for Pediatricians (N=45)

Variable	Beta Wt.
Cluster 3 - Personal control of professional situation	0.4912
Average number of patients seen/week	-0.4
Cluster 6 - Interaction with medical community	0.3018
Sensing - Intuition (Intuitive direction)	0.2934
Length of time in present setting	-0.2517
Extraversion - Introversion (Introverted direction)	0.2221
Thinking - Feeling (Thinking direction)	-0.1598
Cluster 5 - Personal control of income	0.1246
Cluster 1 - Personal patient involvement	0.1215
Judgment - Perception (Judgmental direction)	-0.0719
Cluster 4 - Medical innovation	-0.0625
Cluster 7 - Professional ambition	0.0597
Cluster 2 - Physician - teacher	-0.0298
TOTAL VARIANCE	0.3460

In terms of personality type preferences, those pediatricians who have more introversion, intuition, thinking and judging were more likely to be satisfied than those who have more of the opposite preferences. The sample reflects more introverts, intuitives, feeling and judging types.

Psychiatrists (Tables 20 and 21)

Satisfied psychiatrists are more likely to come from larger communities and practice in larger communities. As for other specialties where it appears, "Assisting other Physicians ... " appears as a source of dissatisfaction, and as might be expected, earning more money is characteristic of the satisfied group. In fact, income is the most important variable in the regression equation (Table 21), followed by the association of satisfaction with working in larger communities. Personality preferences associated with satisfaction for psychiatrists are introversion, sensing, feeling and judgment. This appears surprising in that the psychiatrists in this as well as other samples are predominantly intuitive types. It would appear that satisfaction for these physicians may be enhanced by having an increased amount of sensing available with their predominant preference for intuition. This same phenomenon appears be operating in the results observed for other specialties as well (e. g., general surgery). Thus it may be the case that physicians who appear more "extreme" in their type preferences tend to be more dissatisfied than their perhaps more "differentiated" colleagues of the same type.

Table 20. Psychiatrists N=43 (S=23; D=20)

Variable	Satisfied		Dissatisfied		t	p
	Mean	SD	Mean	SD		
Community size	4.70	0.56	3.90	0.85	3.67	<.01
Pre-college community size	3.43	1.56	2.47	1.43	2.06	<.05
Income	4.00	0.75	3.26	1.33	2.11	<.05
Items rated irrelevant	1.65	1.80	8.10	15.31	2.01	<.05
Items Dr. wants less characteristic	4.09	2.33	8.58	6.14	3.18	<.01
Items Dr. wants more characteristic	12.48	6.16	23.40	14.14	3.36	<.01
Introversion	10.00	6.98	15.15	3.59	2.97	<.01
Extraversion	16.61	7.38	10.30	4.29	3.36	<.01
EI continuous score	114.22	28.52	90.89	15.38	3.20	<.01
Assisting other physicians in performing procedures	1.35	0.94	2.47	1.63	2.76	<.05
Paperwork	5.04	1.02	4.21	2.04	1.72	<.10
Performing habitual or non-varying medical activities	3.09	1.51	3.90	1.63	1.67	<.10
Dealing with patients' emotional difficulties	6.00	0.00	5.42	1.57	1.73	<.10
Availability of consultation services	5.57	0.79	4.72	1.57	2.25	<.05
Maintaining my preferred "pace of life"	3.91	1.53	4.68	1.49	1.64	<.10
Opportunities for spouse to be employed or pursue preferred activities	5.46	1.10	4.68	1.42	1.96	<.10

Table 21. Regression Equation Predicting Satisfaction for Psychiatrists (N=43)

Variable	Beta Wt.
Income	0.4857
Community Size (larger communities)	0.3992
Thinking - Feeling (feeling direction)	0.3466
Cluster 7 - Professional ambition	0.2636
Judgment - Perception (judgmental direction) ·	-0.2591

Sensing - Intuition (sensing direction)	-0.2590
Extraversion - Introversion (Introverted direction)	0.2388
Cluster 1 - Personal patient involvement	0.2121
Cluster 4 - Medical innovation	0.2116
Average number of patients seen/week	-0.1852
Cluster 3 - Personal control of professional situation	0.0984
Cluster 5 - Personal control of income	0.0948
Length of time in present setting	-0.0736
Cluster 6 - Interaction with medical community	0.0131
TOTAL VARIANCE	0.6250

Obstetrics-Gynecology (Tables 22 and 23)

The majority of items differentiating the satisfied and dissatisfied groups appear to reflect style of life factors, as might be expected in a specialty whose hours and demands are relatively unpredictable. Income and its control are also quite important. In fact the regression equation suggests (the sample is one of the smaller ones) that the satisfied physician in this specialty earns a lot, sees fewer patients with whom he has less personal involvement, has more control of his professional activities and has the opportunity for novelty in his practice. Those with more feeling and judgment on the Myers-Briggs are also more likely to be satisfied.

Table 2. Obstetrics-Gynecology N=28 (S=10; D=18)

Variable	Satisfied		Dissatisfied		t	p
	Mean	SD	Mean	SD		
Income	5.00	0.00	4.44	0.62	2.36	<.05
Items Dr. wants more characteristic	16.56	6.13	27.67	7.24	3.94	<.01
Personal control of amount of earnings	4.75	0.71	3.40	1.54	2.37	<.05
Performing therapeutic procedures	5.00	0.00	4.72	0.46	1.79	<.10
Record keeping	4.40	0.84	4.83	0.38	1.88	<.10
Personal control of amount of time devoted to patient care	5.50	0.53	4.39	1.54	2.20	<.05
Working with other physicians on some joint task	5.00	0.50	4.28	1.18	1.75	<.10
Maintaining my preferred "pace of life"	5.10	1.20	2.89	1.57	3.87	<.01
Determining amount of free time and/or						

vacation time	4.80	1.55	3.44	1.65	2.12	<.05
Sufficient time for family and/or outside activities	5.40	0.52	3.00	1.68	4.37	<.01
Sufficient time for family and/or outside activities	5.30	0.95	4.00	1.71	2.20	<.05
Opportunities for spouse to be employed or pursue preferred activities	4.80	1.23	3.40	1.91	2.09	<.05
Cluster 3 Personal control of professional situation	57.79	7.08	42.17	10.33	4.25	<.01

Table 23. - Regression Equation Predicting Satisfaction for Obstetricians-Gynecologists (N•29)

Variable	Beta Wt.
Income	1.2948
Average number of patients seen per week	-0.9591
Thinking-Feeling (Feeling direction)	0.8723
Cluster 1 - Personal patient involvement	-0.8412
Cluster 7 - Professional ambition	0.2099
Cluster 6 - Interaction with medical community	0.1635
Judgment-Perception (Judgment direction)	-0.1324
Cluster 3 - Personal control of professional situation·	0.1141
Cluster 4 - Medical innovation	0.0690
TOTAL VARIANCE	0.9985

Urologists (Tables 24 and 25)

Urologists who see more patients, have been in practice longer, are less highly specialized and have less to do with both their colleagues and the lay public appear more satisfied than those with the opposite characteristics. It is unclear why this particular unusual pattern of variables characterizes urologists. The regression equation indicates that, contrary to expectation and observation of other groups, low professional ambition and lower income are associated with satisfaction for this group.

Table 24. Urologists (N=27 (S=15; D=12)

	Satisfied		Dissatisfied			
	Mean	SD	Mean	SD	t	p
Length of time in present setting	6.93	5.43	3.83	3.54	1.71	<.10
Number of patients seen/week	87.00	41.44	58.33	32.00	1.97	<.10

Items Dr. wants more characteristic	13.57	7.84	24.17	13.57	2.48	<.02
Extraversion	10.33	5.79	15.50	5.07	2.43	<.05
Introversion	16.47	7.27	10.33	4.98	2.49	<.02
EI Continuous score	114.29	26.62	90.67	19.69	2.53	<.02
Focus on a special interest area within a specialty	2.93	1.77	4.22	1.39	1.85	<.10
Intellectual stimulation through interaction with colleagues	4.40	1.35	5.27	0.47	2.04	<.10
Performing diagnostic procedures	4.93	0.26	4.08	1.56	2.08	<.05
Personal control of amount of time devoted to patient care	5.07	1.39	4.00	1.73	1.74	<.10
Opportunity for appreciation and prestige from the lay public	2.93	1.53	4.00	1.09	1.96	<.10
Determining amount of free time and/or vacation time	4.20	1.21	3.20	1.23	2.01	<.10
Cluster 3 - Personal control of professional situation	50.65	7.73	40.51	14.36	2.35	<.05

Other variables in the equation appear in the direction one would expect. e. g. clusters 4, 2, 6 and 3. It appears likely that a variable such as practice organization may influence satisfaction relationships for this sample. Relationships to satisfaction of particular variables should therefore not be considered as necessarily direct but may be the result of some intervening variable which is not available for examination. It is primarily the association of satisfaction with increased feeling which does not correspond to the predominance of preferences for this group.

Table 25. Regression Equation Predicting Satisfaction for Urologists (N=29)

Variable	Beta Wt.
Cluster 7 - Professional ambition	-0.7792
Income	-0.5654
Length of time in present setting	0.4067
Cluster 4 - Medical Innovation	0.3901
Cluster 2 - Physician - Teacher	0.3829
Judgment.- Perception (Judgmental direction)	-0.3490
Cluster 6 ~ Interaction with medical community	0.3064
Thinking - Feeling (Feeling direction)	0.3013

Extraversion - Introversion (Introverted direction)	0.2549
Cluster 3. - Personal control of professional situation	0.2230
Average number of patients seen per week	0.1913
Sensing - Intuition (Intuitive direction)	0.0644
Cluster 1 - Personal patient involvement	0.0419
TOTAL VARIANCE	0.7268

Orthopedic Surgeons (Tables 26 and 27)

As for psychiatrists and obstetricians, amount of income and its control are important to orthopedic surgeons, as are life style factors in this specialty which is often associated with large patient loads. Like for obstetricians, the regression equation indicates that seeing fewer patients and having less personal involvement with them, leads to satisfaction as does more recent graduation from medical school. Higher introversion, sensing, feeling and judgment are sources of satisfaction for these physicians. This is notable in that the sample contains more than twice as many thinking as feeling types.

Table 26. Orthopedic Surgeons N=37 (S=19; D=18)

	Satisfied		Dissatisfied			
	Mean	SD	Mean	SD	t	p
Income	4.94	0.24	4.00	1.11	3.41	<.01
Items rated irrelevant	0.79	1.81	2.61	4.10	1.76	<.10
Items Dr. wants less characteristic	7.06	4.95	11.83	5.22	2.81	<.01
Items Dr. wants more characteristic	12.78	7.11	30.89	8.60	6.89	<.01
(Illegible term)	5.63	0.68	5.00	1.33	1.83	<.10
Personal control of amount of earnings	4.42	1.61	2.83	1.86	2.78	<.01
Access to hospital facilities	5.74	0.45	4.78	1.73	2.33	<.05
Responsibility for defining one's role, duties and activities	5.35	0.70	4.65	1.54	1.72	<.10
Personal control of amount of time devoted to patient care	4.67	1.33	3.77	1.39	1.96	<.10
Access to new developments in a field of interest or specialization	5.10	0.99	4.22	1.40	2.23	<.05
Opportunity for appreciation and prestige from the lay public	4.68	1.00	3.28	1.81	2.95	<.01

Maintaining my preferred pace of life	4.67	1.19	3.78	1.35	2.09	<.05
Determining amount of free time and/or vacation time	4.61	1.09	3.56	1.42	2.50	<.05
Opportunities for spouse to be employed or pursue preferred activities	5.00	1.28	3.94	1.83	1.97	<.10
Cluster 6: Interaction with the medical community	55.48	4.21	48.56	10.46	2.67	<.05

Table 27. Regression Equation Predicting Satisfaction for Orthopedic Surgeons (N•38)

Variable	Beta Wt.
Income	0.9823
Cluster 5 .. Personal Control of Income	-0.8054
Year of graduation from medical school	0.6682
Sensing - intuition (Sensing direction)	-0.5683
Cluster 6 - Interaction with medical community	0.3325
Cluster 1 - Personal patient involvement	-0.3306
Cluster 7 - Professional ambition	0.2918
Judgment - Perception (Judgmental direction)	-0.2064
Average. number of patients seen per week .	-0.1812
Cluster 2 .. Physician-Teacher	0.1779
Extraversion - Introversion (Introverted direction)	0.0597
Thinking ... Feeling (Feeling direction)	0.0348
TOTAL VARIANCE	0.5927

Anesthesiologists (Tables 28 and 29)

The t-test table for this group appears to be a more extreme example of that obtained for pediatricians in that only four items significantly differed for the two groups. The satisfied anesthesiologists in this analysis appear able to provide patient care outside of their usual setting and work less often with paraprofessionals than their dissatisfied colleagues. The regression equation is interesting in that it is one of the two (Ophthalmologists being the second) in which a type variable leads the regression equation. Further, the type distribution for this sample indicates that 77% are introverts with 23% extraverts. Thus, it appears that those anesthesiologists who have available a greater amount of extraversion in their predominantly introverted personalities, have a greater .opportunity for satisfaction. The other three preferences also contribute to satisfaction for this group.

Seeing fewer patients is associated with satisfaction which may be related to the association of lower income with satisfaction. It is puzzling, however, to find that satisfaction is associated with decreased personal control of the professional situation. This does not occur for any other specialty and must be assumed to be a function of some practice characteristic or specialty characteristic which serves as an intervening variable in relation to this cluster of items.

Table 28. Anesthesiologists N=31 (S=15; D=16)

	Satisfied		Dissatisfied		
Variable	Mean	SD	Mean	SD	t
Items Dr. wants more characteristic	13.07	13.69	22.81	9.43	2.29
Working with paraprofessionals or physician-extenders	3.60	2.13	5.39	1.12	2.70
Referring patients to other practitioners or institutions	2.07	1.54	1.31	0.70	1.77
Providing some form of patient care outside of the major practice setting (e.g., community clinics, hospitals, etc.)	1.87	1.19	1.00	0.00	2.92

Table 29. Regression Equation Predicting Satisfaction for Anesthesiologists (N•32)

Variable	Beta Wt.
Extraversion - Introversion- (Extraverted direction)	-0.9958
Income	-0.7748
Average number of patients seen per week	-0.7184
Cluster 6 - Interaction with medical community	0.5811
Cluster 3 - Personal control of professional situation	-0.5500
Sensing - Intuition (Sensing direction)	-0.4841
Judgment - Perception (Judgment direction)	-0.4041
Community size (smaller communities)	-0.3696
Cluster 7.- Professional ambition	-0.3666
Cluster 2 - Physician-Teacher	0.2389
Cluster 5 - Interaction with medical community	0.2378
Year of graduation from medical school	0.1960
Cluster 4 - Medical innovation	0.1284
Thinking - Feeling (Thinking direction)	-0.0812
Cluster 1 - Personal patient involvement	-0.0690
TOTAL VARIANCE	0.6215

Internists (Table 30 and 31)

Notable about the table of t-tests for internists is its contrast to the preceding table for anesthesiologists with regard to the numbers of variables discriminating the satisfied and dissatisfied groups. In this respect it is similar to the table for the total sample, which would be as long as this if items contained in the seven clusters had been included. It would appear then that internal medicine as a specialty is characterized by a great amount of variability in the way it may be practiced. This would appear reasonable in light of the wide range of patient populations addressed, focused on a variety of patient problems and the possibility of practicing the specialty in any kind of practice organization.

As might be expected, satisfied internists have greater control over their professional lives, interact more with colleagues and students, and see greater challenges in their practices. The regression equation shows that lower income is associated with satisfaction. This most likely is a function of the association between shorter time in the present setting and more recent graduation from medical school with satisfaction. Internists who have practiced a shorter period of time are probably also earning less money than their elder colleagues. It is interesting, however. that increased income does not appear to automatically increase satisfaction for internists. It might be the case that higher income is achieved at the cost of lessened ability to control the professional situation (Cluster 3), which is almost invariably associated with dissatisfaction for physicians in general.

Personality type relationships are not particularly notable for this sample, although the sample contains slightly more extraverts than introverts.

Table 30. Internists N=39 (S=19; D=20)

Variable	Satisfied		Dissatisfied			
	Mean	SD	Mean	SD	t	p
Items rated irrelevant	1.16	1.46	8.95	12.89	2.62	<.025
Items Dr. wants less characteristic	4.90	3.03	9.16	4.98	3.19	<.005
Items Dr. wants more characteristic	8.67	5.72	26.25	11.30	5.95	<.005
Dealing with ethical or moral issues in the practice of medicine	5.00	1.00	3.65	1.84	2.82	<.005
Assisting other physicians in performing procedures	2.11	1.37	3.15	1.53	2.24	<.025
Working with paraprofessionals or physician extenders	3.61	1.24	4.47	1.19	2.01	<.05
Maintaining a fairly consistent and predictable patient-scheduling system	5.11	1.37	4.06	1.83	1.98	<.05
Dealing with emergency medical problems	4.53	0.91	4.05	1.32	1.31	<.10
Access to hospital facilities	5.90	0.32	5.05	1.54	2.35	<.025
Opportunity for affiliation with a medical school	4.78	1.87	3.45	2.28	1.95	<.05
Opportunity for professional advancement	5.11	0.74	3.79	1.84	2.89	<.005
Teaching medical students, interns or residents	4.89	1.61	3.95	2.01	1.58	<.10

Intellectual stimulation through interaction with colleagues	5.58	0.77	4.75	1.12	2.68	<.025
Performing therapeutic procedures	1.63	1.30	2.68	1.73	2.12	<.025
Dealing with new or unusual patient problems	5.16	0.69	3.90	1.65	3.08	<.005
Performing diagnostic procedures	2.90	1.76	3.75	1.55	1.62	<..10
Satisfactory coverage for patients during periods of absence	5.90	0.32	4.42	1.71	3.69	<.005
Testifying in court in medical-legal proceedings	1.42	0.51	1.80	0.89	1.62	<.10
Responsibility for defining one's role, duties and activities	4.94	1.44	4.11	1.97	1.51	<.10
Personal control over amount of time devoted to patient care	5.28	0.96	4.26	1.56	2.37	<.025
Supervision of subordinates	5.16	1.12	4.32	1.60	1.90	<.05
Trying out new ideas	5.11	0.88	3.95	1.50	2.91	<.005
Expanding one's own knowledge in an area of medicine	5.42	0.90	4.42	1.43	2.58	<.025
Financial constraints limiting provision of patient care	2.11	1.52	3.30	1.84	2.20	<.025
Working with other physicians on some joint task	5.11	0.74	3.80	1.73	3.03	<.005
Access to new developments in a field of interest or specialization	5.00	0.82	4.10	1.52	2.29	<.025
Sharing patient responsibility with other physicians	5.37	0.68	4.15	1.57	3.12	<.005
Availability of consultation services	5.95	0.23	4.95	1.47	2.93	<.005
Isolation from other physicians	1.37	0.76	3.10	1.59	1.89	<.05
Opportunity for prestige and recognition from colleagues	5.00	0.75	4.30	1.59	1.74	<.05
Determining amount of free time and/or	4.21	1.27	3.35	1.63	1.83	<.05

vacation time						
Sufficient time for family and/or outside activities	4.11	1.24	3.30	1.59	1.75	<.05
Cultural or recreational activities in my geographical area	4.90	0.99	3.90	1.62	2.30	<.025
Availability of desirable public school system	5.39	0.78	3.60	1.90	3.72	<.005
Opportunities for spouse to be employed or pursue preferred activities	5.31	1.01	3.60	1.79	3.41	<.005
Active participation in non-medical community affairs	4.67	1,14	3.35	1.57	2.94	<.005
Opportunity to follow and evaluate patient progress	5.47	0.70	4.80	1.51	1.77	<.05
Cluster 3: Personal control of professional situation	50.47	9.01	43.97	9.48	2.30	<.025
Cluster 4: Medical Innovation	56.30	7.43	43.67	14.98	3.31	<.005
Cluster 6: Interaction with medical community	56.61	3.81	47.07	11.56	3.42	<.005
Cluster 7: Professional prestige	56.73	6.47	48.65	11.97	2.60	<.025

Table 31 - Regression Equation Predicting Satisfaction for Internists (N=40)

Variable	Beta Wt.
Income	-0.4937
Cluster 3 - Personal control of professional situation	0.3750
Cluster 5 - Personal control of income	0.3184
Thinking - Feeling (Feeling direction)	0.2967
Year since graduation from medical school	-0.2792
Cluster 7 • Professional ambition	0.2553
Cluster 4 - Medical innovation	0.2071
Length of time in present setting	-0.1555
Community size (larger communities)	0.0985
Extraversion - Introversion (Extraverted direction)	-0.0753
TOTAL VARIANCE	0.5442

General Surgeons (Tables 32 and 33)

Satisfied general surgeons are characterized by having greater opportunity to interact with and achieve recognition from their professional colleagues. Those who work alone, are isolated and have less opportunity to consult with colleagues are in the dissatisfied group. Although the predominant types in the sample are sensing, thinking and judging, it appears that those who have less of each of these preferences are more satisfied than those with stronger preferences. The regression equation shows this same relationship to satisfaction for judgment-perception, as well as for extraversion. Introverts predominate in the sample. It is also interesting that although increased income leads to satisfaction for the group, decreased personal control of income is the most important variable predictive of satisfaction. In addition, seeing more patients but having less personal involvement with them, contributes to satisfaction.

Table 32. General Surgeons N=27 (S=13; D=14)

Variable	Satisfied		Dissatisfied			
	Mean	SD	Mean	SD	t	p
Income	4.20	1.03	3.33	1.15	1.84	<.10
Items Dr. wants less characteristic	5.08	2.07	10.00	5.94	2.72	<.02
Items Dr. wants more characteristic	13.15	7.73	26.50	12.28	3.34	<.01
Introversion Myers-Briggs	11.69	10.22	20.29	9.39	2.27	<.05
Extraversion Myers-Briggs	8.00	4.90	11.86	6.36	1.75	<.10
Perception Myers-Briggs ?	13.54	7.25	18.43	7.10	1.77	<.10
Intellectual stimulation through interaction with colleagues	5.62	0.65	4.69	1.38	2.18	<.05
Working alone	1.54	0.78	2.92	1.71		<.02
Case consultation with other professional personnel	4.92	0.29	4.54	0.66	1.82	<.10
Testifying in court in medical-legal proceedings	1.46	0.66	1.92	0.52	1.91	<.10
Trying out new ideas	4.85	1.07	3.92	1.55	1.77	<.10
Working with other physicians on some joint task	5.08	1.32	4.08	1.32	1.93	<.10
Access to new developments in a field of interest or specialization	5.31	1.11	4.31	1.44	1.99	<.10
Isolation from other physicians	1.00	0.00	2.39	1.81	2.65	<.02

Opportunity for prestige and recognition from colleagues	5.54	0.52	4.31	1.44	2.91	<.01
Cultural or recreational activities in my geographical area	5.31	0.86	4.31	1.55	2.04	<.10
Opportunities for spouse to be employed or pursue preferred activities	5.31	0.95	4.15	1.91	1.95	<.10
Medical innovation	56.03	9.15	44.38	16.80	0.21	<.05

Table 33. Regression Equation Predicting Satisfaction for General Surgeons (N=27)

Variable	Beta Wt.
Cluster 5 - Personal control of income	-3.9152
Average number of patients seen per week	3.3092
Income	2.9555
Cluster 7 - Professional ambition	2.5882
Cluster 1 - Personal patient involvement	-2.1547
Judgment - Perception (Perceptive direction)	1.5068
Extraversion - Introversion (Extraverted direction)	-1.2891
Cluster 2 - Physician-Teacher	1.1553
Community size (larger communities)	0.6902
Cluster 6 - Interaction with medical community	-0.5370
Cluster 3 - Personal control of professional situation	0.1403
TOTAL VARIANCE	0.9870

Pathologists (Tables 34 and 35)

Satisfied pathologists were raised in smaller communities and have a greater opportunity for interaction and prestige from the medical community. Performing therapeutic procedures and referring patients are sources of satisfaction for them as is the small amount of personal patient involvement characteristic of their practices. It appears that pathologists would prefer to have less than minimal patient involvement.

The regression equation shows that professional ambition, being in their setting a longer time, lack of focus on medical innovation and less teaching, are major sources of satisfaction. For most other groups, a shorter time in the setting, and greater opportunity for innovation as well as teaching, are associated with satisfaction. Greater intuition and perception contribute to satisfaction in spite of the type distribution which is characterized by a large majority of sensing-judging types.

Table 34. Pathologists N=49 (S=29; D=20)

Variable	Satisfied		Dissatisfied			
	Mean	SD	Mean	SD	t	p
Pre-college community size	2.66	1.59	3.45	1.57	1.73	<.10
Income	4.48	0.85	4.00	1.05	1.71	<.10
Items Dr. wants less characteristic	4.25	3.91	10.80	8.48	3.60	<.01
Items Dr. wants more characteristic	9.93	5.72	21.89	10.92	4.81	<.01
Intellectual stimulation through interaction with colleagues	4.59	1.40	5.44	0.98	2.27	<.05
Performing therapeutic procedures	1.19	0.69	2.39	1.85	3.01	<.01
Referring patients to other practitioners or institutions	1.79	1.23	2.72	1.71	2.16	<.05
Sufficient time for family and/or outside activities	4.79	1.29	3.84	1.89	2.07	<.05
Availability of desirable public school system	5.32	0.86	4.47	1.81	2.15	<.05
Active participation in non-medical community affairs	3.97	1.55	2.74	1.59	2.66	<.02
Cluster 1 Personal patient involvement	30.03	8.54	35.44	9.67	2.07	<.05
Cluster 3 Personal control of professional situation	54.45	8.00	46.71	16.31	2.21	<.05
Cluster 7 Professional prestige	54.88	7.19	48.38	15.04	2.02	<.05

Table 35. Regression Equation Predicting Satisfaction for Pathologists (N=50)

Variable	Beta Wt.
Cluster 7 - Professional ambition	0.5125
Length of time in present setting	0.4735
Cluster 4 Medical innovation	-0.4643
Cluster 2 - Physician-Teacher	-0.2729
Cluster 5 - Personal control of income	0.2610
Cluster 6 - Interaction with medical community	0.2239
Year of graduation from medical school	0.1907
Cluster 3 - Personal control of professional situation	0.1701
Judgment - Perception (Perceptive direction)	0.1352

Sensing - Intuition (Intuitive direction)		0.0891
TOTAL VARIANCE		0.4651

Radiologists: (Tables 36 and 37)

Important sources of satisfaction for radiologists are variables concerning life style, as well as interaction with and availability of other health professionals. Unlike pathologists, a shorter time in the present setting is associated with satisfaction. The negative association of cluster 5-Personal Control of Income is most likely related to typical practice organizations of radiologists, which as a referral specialty probably permit a minimum of such personal control. Practice styles which permit such control would be unusual and may have other features which are more directly related to dissatisfaction. In terms of personality type preferences, those radiologists with greater extraversion, sensing, feeling and judging are more satisfied, while the sample contains more introverts, and nearly twice as many thinking as feeling types.

Table 36. Radiologists N=24 (S=15; D=9)

Variable	Satisfied Mean	SD	Dissatisfied Mean	SD	t	p
Items Dr. wants less characteristic	5.40	3.54	11.44	10.04	2.15	<.05
Items Dr. wants more characteristic	13.00	5.62	22.33	10.17	2.85	<.01
Feeling Myers-Briggs	9.60	5.91	5.67	4.27	1.74	<.01
Assisting other physicians in performing procedures	3.33	1.35	4.43	0.54	2.06	<.10
Dealing with emergency medical problems	3.27	1.16	2.38	1.19	1.74	<.10
Opportunity for affiliation with a medical school	4.33	2.02	2.50	2.14	2.03	<.10
Teaching medical students, interns or residents	4.27	2.05	2.75	1.75	1.77	<.10
Performing habitual or non-varying medical activities	3.80	1.37	5.00	0.93	2.21	<.05
Responsibility for defining one's role, duties and activities	5.27	0.88	4.63	0.74	1.75	<.10
Personal control of amount of time devoted to patient care	5.13	0.74	3.38	1.85	3.27	<.01
Supervision of subordinates	5.67	0.62	4.63	1.69	2.17	<.05

Dealing with patients' emotional difficulties	1.77	1.67	1.00	0.00	1.85	<.10
Availability of consultation services	5.67	0.49	5.13	0.99	1.77	<.10
Working with or under a community board or citizens' group	1.53	0.83	3.13	2.36	2.40	<.05
Maintaining my preferred "pace of life"	4.60	1.72	3.00	1.31	2.29	<.05
Determining amount of free time and/or vacation time	4.33	2.02	2.88	1.73	1.73	<.10
Sufficient time for family and/or outside activities	5.20	1.08	3.50	1.51	3.13	<.01
Cultural or recreational activities in my geographical area	5.20	1.27	3.88	1.73	2.11	<.05
Cluster 2 Physician Teacher	54.88	7.43	44.58	18.07	1.97	<.10
Cluster 3 Personal control of professional situation	55.08	8.47	37.27	17.08	3.43	<.01
Cluster 6 Interaction with the medical community	47.69	5.75	37.18	18.16	2.09	<.05

Table 37. Regression Equation Predicting Satisfaction for Radiologists (N=25)

Variable	Beta Wt.
Cluster 3 - Personal control of professional situation	0.7461
Extraversion - Introversion (Extraverted direction)	-0.5685
Length of time in present setting	-0.4156
Cluster 5 - Personal control of income	-0.4239
Sensing - Intuition (Sensing direction)	-0.2708
Judgment - Perception (Judgmental direction)	-0.2349
Thinking - Feeling (Feeling direction)	0.2177
Cluster 6 - Interaction with medical community	-0.1600
Cluster 2 - Physician-Teacher	0.0996
Year of graduation from medical school	0.0915
Cluster 4 - Medical innovation	0.0610
TOTAL VARIANCE	0.6584

Ophthalmologists (Table 38 and 39)

Satisfied ophthalmologists see a greater number of patients and have greater control over life style factors. The regression equation indicates that they are one of the two specialties where a type variable is most important to satisfaction. In fact, the first three variables in the equation are type variables. Those physicians who are higher on intuition, feeling and judgment are more satisfied. The type distribution for this sample, though predominantly judging, contains a fairly even distribution for sensing-intuition and thinking-feeling. Like pathologists ophthalmologists are more satisfied with less opportunity for medical innovation. The same is true for interacting with other health professionals.

Table 38. Ophthalmologists N=26 (S=12; D=14)

Variable	Satisfied Mean	SD	Dissatisfied Mean	SD	t	p
Pre-college community size	3.58	1.38	2.57	1.40	1.85	<.10
Number of patients seen per week	153.00	53.57	103.92	50.71	2.30	<.05
Items Dr. wants less characteristic	7.50	4.25	14.55	7.34	2.85	<.01
Items Dr. wants more characteristic	10.64	7.71	28.07	7.90	5.53	<.01
Intuition Myers-Briggs	13.58	6.43	9.50	5.27	1.73	<.10
SN continuous score	115.00	23.79	92.93	32.46	1.95	<.10
Feeling Myers-Briggs	19.00	6.25	14.00	7.06	1.90	<.10
Working alone	2.33	1.78	4.14	1.88	2.51	<.02
Organizational administration (e. g., committee work, policy development)	3.92	0.90	2.86	1.41	2.24	<.05
Performing diagnostic procedures	3.00	1.65	1.71	1.27	2.24	<.05
Delegation of certain medical tasks to subordinates	4.58	1.56	3.21	1.63	2.18	<.05
Satisfactory coverage for patients during periods of absence	5.92	0.29	4.29	1.38	4.00	<.01
Supervision and/or teaching medical students or medical personnel (e. g., para- medics)	3.67	1.23	2.57	1.60	1.93	<.10
Availability of consultation services	5.75	0.45	4.93	1.14	2.34	<.05
Opportunity for prestige and recognition from						

colleagues	5.00	1.41	3.86	1.56	1.94	<.10
Maintaining my preferred pace of life	4.92	1.08	3.64	1.69	2.24	<.05
Determining amount of free time and/or vacation time	5.42	1.00	3.86	1.35	3.30	<.01
Sufficient time for family and/or outside activities	4.67	1.44	3.42	1.83	1.86	<.10
Cultural or recreational activities in my geographical area	5.25	0.87	4.00	1.53	2.49	<.02
Active participation in non-medical community affairs	4.67	1.44	2.43	1.34	4.11	<.01
Opportunity to follow and evaluate patient progress	5.83	0.39	5.07	0.83	2.91	<.01
Cluster 3 Personal control of professional situation	57.09	7.33	45.87	11.20	2.94	<.01

Table 39. Regression Equation Predicting Satisfaction for Ophthalmologists (N=26)

Variable	Beta Wt.
Judgment - Perception (Judgmental direction).	-0.6037
Sensing - Intuition (Intuitive direction)	0.5600
Thinking - Feeling (Feeling direction)	0.4067
Cluster 7 - Professional ambition	0.3922
Cluster 6 - Interaction with medical community	-0.1332
Cluster 4 - Medical innovation	-0.1062
Cluster 1 - Personal patient involvement	0.0941
Cluster 2 - Physician-Teacher	0.0514
TOTAL VARIANCE	0.5414

General Practitioners (Tables 40 and 41)

Satisfied GPs are highly involved with patients as well as with their colleagues. They appear to have greater opportunity to vary their activities and gain satisfaction from supervision and teaching. They have a greater opportunity to pursue innovation in medicine as well as maintain continuity of care for their patients. The regression equation indicates that interacting with the medical community is most important to satisfaction with increased professional ambition a source of satisfaction. Like most other groups, a shorter time in the setting and seeing fewer patients leads to satisfaction.

Those who have greater extraversion, sensing, and feeling are more satisfied. This is in line with the preponderance of types in the distribution.

Table 40. General Practitioners N=29 (S=15; D=14)

Variable	Satisfied		Dissatisfied			
	Mean	SD	Mean	SD	t	p
Items Dr. wants more characteristic	12.54	6.63	27.36	13.29	3.62	0.01
Extraversion on Myers-Briggs	15.40	4.81	10.50	6.98	2.21	<.05
Introversion on Myers-Briggs	9.53	3.98	16.14	7.79	2.91	<.01
EI Continuous score	89.27	15.85	112.29	29.38	2.65	<.02
Dealing with emergency medical problems	5.13	0.95	4.23	1.48	1.92	<.10
Working alone	2.00	1.41	3.46	1.66	2.51	<.02
Delegating of certain medical tasks to subordinates	5.00	0.93	4.15	1.57	1.76	<.10
Teaching medical students, interns or residents	2.93	1.53	1.86	1.17	2.11	<.05
Providing some form of patient care outside of the major practice setting (e. g., community clinics, hospitals, etc.)	3.40	1.45	1.50	1.29	3.72	<.01
Explaining diagnoses and treatment plans to patients and their families	5.00	0.00	4.79	0.43	1.88	<.10
Personal control of amount of time devoted to patient care	5.20	0.94	4.31	1.18	2.22	<.05
Sharing patient responsibility with other physicians	4.93	0.92	3.85	1.63	2.15	<.05
Sharing doubts, frustrations or problems with colleagues	4.67	1.35	3.42	1.73	2.11	<.05
Direct patient contact	6.00	0.00	5.54	0.66	2.72	<.02
Opportunities for spouse to be employed or pursue preferred activities	5.07	1.33	3.69	1.75	2.32	<.05
Opportunity to follow and evaluate patient progress	5.60	0.51	4.77	1.01	2.80	<.01
Cluster 1 Personal patient involvement	56.86	2.59	53.85	3.92	2.46	<.02

Cluster 3 Personal control of professional situation	53.90	7.79	44.93	15.93	1.95	<.10
Cluster 4 Medical innovation	48.86	8.32	39.99	15.98	1.90	<.10
Cluster 6 Interaction with the medical community	51.55	7.79	42.23	15.30	2.09	<.05

Table 41. Regression Equation Predicting Satisfaction for General Practitioners (N•29)

Variable	Beta Wt.
Cluster 6 - Interaction with medical community	0.6181
Cluster 7 - Professional ambition	-0.5667
Sensing - Intuition (Sensing direction)	-0.4797
Extraversion - Introversion (Extraverted direction)	-0.3959
Community size (smaller communities)	-0.3952
Income	0.3138
Cluster 2 – Physician-Teacher	0.3452
Thinking - Feeling (Feeling direction)	0.2345
Cluster 4 - Medical innovation	0.2196
Cluster 3 - Personal control of professional situation	0.1686
Average number of patients seen per week	-0.1512
Length of time in present setting	-0.1030
Cluster 5 - Personal control of income	-0.0756
Cluster I - Personal patient involvement	0.0525
TOTAL VARIANCE	0.6780

Family Practitioners (Tables 42 and 43)

Some interesting differences in the patterns of satisfactions are evident for FPs as compared to GPs. Dealing with emergency medical problems is characteristic of the satisfied GP's and of the dissatisfied FPs. Dealing with ethical or moral issues in the practice of medicine, seems to be a predominant factor in relation to satisfaction. In the regression equation, the most important source of satisfaction is cluster 4, Medical innovation, followed by cluster 2 -Physician Teacher. Personal control of income (cluster 5) is also important, while for GPs it has a negative relation to satisfaction.

In terms of personality type, satisfaction for FPs is associated with greater extraversion, thinking and Judging. Sensing-Intuition appears to be related to satisfaction. Thus the FPs differ from the GPs in personality type - satisfaction relationships, particularly in that apparently the GPs satisfaction is increased by having increased feeling, and the FPs by having greater thinking on the Myers-Briggs.

Table 42. Family Practice N=44 (S=21; D=23)

Variable	Satisfied		Dissatisfied		t	p
	Mean	SD	Mean	SD		
Pre-college community size	3.24	1.51	2.13	1.39	2.53	<.05
Amount of time in present setting	7.38	6.04	12.00	8.31	2.09	<.05
Items Dr. wants less characteristic	3.70	2.72	12.70	6.09	6.04	<.01
Items Dr. wants more characteristic	9.15	5.31	20.48	6.80	6.02	<.01
Year of graduation from medical school	57.33	5.50	53.17	5.06	2.61	<.05
Illegible (unknown variable)	42.63	6.45	49.09	4.83	3.49	<.01
Extraversion on Myers-Briggs	14.14	7.10	9.44	5.97	2.39	<.05
Introversion on Myers-Briggs	12.52	7.82	16.65	6.56	1.90	<.10
EI Continuous score	97.76	29.72	116.18	25.23	2.19	<.05
Dealing with ethical or moral issues in the practice of medicine	4.76	1.34	4.00	1.41	1.81	<.10
Reading journals and medical books	4.67	0.48	4.34	0.65	1.84	<.10
Dealing with emergency medical problems	5.05	1.12	5.44	1.04	1.89	<.10
Opportunity for affiliation with a medical school	4.48	1.94	2.35	1.82	3.75	<.01
Teaching medical students, interns or residents	3.81	1.99	2.22	1.70	2.86	<.01
Performing habitual or non-varying medical activities	3.57	1.57	4.74	1.21	2.78	<.01
Devoting time to particular patient problems or kinds of patients	4.43	1.60	3.55	1.68	1.76	<.10
Responsibility for defining one's role, duties and activities	5.33	0.97	4.52	1.59	2.02	<.05
Personal control of amount of time devoted to patient care	5.09	0.94	3.96	1.82	2.57	<.05
Delegating some medical tasks to subordinates	5.38	0.74	4.35	2.69	2.69	<.01

Trying out new ideas	4.67	1.07	3.73	1.35	2.52	<.05
Expanding one's own knowledge in an area of medicine	5.33	0.86	4.57	1.08	2.60	<.05
Access to new developments in a field of interest or specialization	4.90	1.12	4.05	1.36	2.21	<.05
Opportunity for appreciation and prestige from the lay public	4.65	1.50	3.48	1.78	2.28	<.05
Cluster 2 Physician Teacher	48.79	11.28	40.69	6.96	2.89	<.01
Cluster 3 Personal control of the professional situation	52.11	12.13	45.02	11.04	2.03	<.05
Cluster 4 Medical innovation	53.07	7.66	44.25	7.92	3.75	<.01
Cluster 7 Professional ambition	49.54	9.84	44.60	9.04	1.74	<.10

Table 43. Regression Equation Predicting Satisfaction for Family Practitioners (N=45)

Variable	Beta Wt.
Cluster 4 - Medical innovation	0.4575
Cluster 2 - Physician - Teacher	0.4389
Cluster 5 - Personal control of income	0.3612
Extraversion - Introversion (Extraverted direction)	-0.3533
Judgment - Perception (Judgmental direction)	0.0000
Cluster 7 - Professional ambition	-0.1138
Cluster 1 - Personal patient involvement	-0.2105
Average number of patients seen per week	-0.1960
Thinking - Feeling (Thinking direction)	-0.1831
Length of time in present setting	-0.1766
Cluster 3 - Personal control of professional situation	0.1584
Cluster 6 - Interaction with medical community	-0.1196
TOTAL VARIANCE	0.65

Summary of satisfaction for specialties

The large number of variables examined and the different analyses finding sometimes different results, make a comprehensive understanding of these data somewhat difficult. It is evident that some variables are unimportant for any group, others idiosyncratic to one or two groups, and others occur for a number of groups. In terms of variables which appear to be of importance to satisfaction for 5 or more groups, the following occur:

Personal control of amount of time devoted to patient care (8 groups)

Cultural or recreational activities in my geographic area (8 groups)
Opportunities for spouse to be employed or pursue preferred activities (8 groups)
Cluster 3-Personal Control of the Professional Situation (8 groups)
Determining amount of free time or vacation time (7 groups)
Income (6 groups)
Maintaining my preferred pace of life (6 groups)
Sufficient time for family and outside activities (6 groups)
Pre-college community size (5 groups)
Responsibility for defining one's role, duties and activities (5 groups)
Access to new developments in a field of interest or specialization (5 groups)
Dealing with emergency medical problems (5 groups)
Intellectual stimulation through interaction with colleagues (5 groups)
Accessibility of consultation services (5 groups)
Opportunity for prestige and recognition from colleagues (5 groups)
Cluster 4 - Medical Innovation (5 groups)
Cluster 6 - Interaction with the Medical Community (5 groups)
Cluster 7 - Professional Prestige (5 groups)

These more frequently appearing variables would seem to reflect a set of factors that are of general importance to career satisfaction across a number of different specialties and/or for physicians in general. Though the direction of differences sometimes varies with a particular variable it may be assumed that a consideration of the above factors is worthwhile in attempting to maximize physician satisfaction regardless of the specialty involved. Where concern is with a particular specialty, these kinds of data provide some empirical evidence directing attention to specific sources of satisfaction or dissatisfaction. A source of satisfaction for one specialty may be a source of dissatisfaction for another. This suggests that more discriminating approaches may need to be taken in order to satisfy the career needs of different kinds of physicians.

Addendum: Family Practice Teachers and Residents

Myers-Briggs Type Indicator responses were compared in a "fortuitous" sample of 85 residents in ten different family practice programs to those of 91 program directors and teachers who attended the 1973 American Association of Family Practice meeting in Kansas City [78]. Although both samples had a relatively large number of sensing-judging types (44 percent for teachers and 52 percent for residents) the sample of teachers had a wider representation of the types, with more falling into the intuitive category and fewer into the sensing category. Both teachers and residents differed from other samples of physicians in their greater proportion of sensing-judging types but the teachers included a broader representation of the 16 types than did the residents due to more intuitive-feeling types. It was concluded that:

> program directors and teachers value imagination, inspiration and possibilities as indicated by their preference for intuition as a mode of perception. Residents, in contrast, perceive more often via sensing, and thus tend to be more realistic,

practical, and observant. In addition, in making judgments, teachers tend to use personal values as a criterion (feeling preferences) while residents prefer impersonal logic as a basis for their judgments (thinking preference). A sensing-thinking type resident in a patient care situation would tend to focus on accumulating facts about the patient and handle these facts with impersonal analysis. He would be seen as practical and matter-of-fact in dealing with patients. In contrast, his intuitive- feeling teacher might focus his attention on the possibilities inherent in the patient care situation and relate to the patient with more personal warmth. He would be seen as dealing with patients in an enthusiastic and sensitive fashion.

It was noted that the psychological types being attracted to family medicine tend to be under-represented among medical students and may be more inclined to practice family medicine rather than teach it. She wondered whether or not the different types represented in the family practice faculty might eventually influence the types who are drawn to that specialty in the future.

7 SOURCES OF SATISFACTION FOR PRACTICE ORGANIZATIONS

Naomi Quenk, PhD

This chapter continues analysis of the sample of physicians described in the previous chapter but with a focus on work-settings or practice organizations.

Data analyses for practice organizations omit analyses for certain combinations of practice organizations. In some instances t-tests, were performed for combined practice organizations but no regression equation was deemed appropriate because a large amount of intra-group variability was hypothesized. In other cases, only regression equations are presented because the particular subgroup had already been included in a t-test analysis of a combination of practice organizations. Analyses of most single institutional practice organizations were omitted due to the small numbers of cases available.

Private Practice (solo, partnerships, small and large groups) (Table 44)

For physicians in private practice, regardless of specialty area, important sources of satisfaction appear to involve a variety of life style factors, professional independence, intellectual challenge, and recognition by both colleagues and the lay public. Dissatisfaction is associated with working alone, working with paraprofessionals and working with other physicians in the capacity of assistant. The two clusters which do not discriminate satisfied from dissatisfied private practitioners are Personal Patient Involvement, which may be assumed to be high in general in this practice setting, and Physician-Teacher, which is relatively uncharacteristic of these physicians. There are no discriminating personality type variables, probably due to the diversity of specialists included.

Table 44. Private Practice (all forms) N=290 (s=152; D=138)

	Satisfied		Dissatisfied			
Variable	Mean	SD	Mean	SD	t	p
Pre-college community size	3.03	1.50	2.49	1.47	3.05	<.002
Income	4.50	0.85	4.26	0.93	2.23	<.027
Items rated irrelevant	1.95	3.13	4.84	9.23	3.41	<.001
Items Dr. wants less characteristic	5.49	3.91	11.25	6.34	8.57	<.000
Items Dr. wants more characteristic	11.78	5.96	26.55	10.64	14.24	<.000
Assisting other physicians in performing medical tasks	3.11	1.46	3.44	1.42	1.93	<.055
Working with paraprofessionals or physician-extenders	3.77	1.63	4.24	1.48	2.32	<.021
Maintaining a fairly consistent and predictable patient-scheduling system	4.81	1.44	4.26	1.69	2.79	<.006
Personal control of amount of earnings	4.48	1.51	3.75	1.71	3.77	<.000
Access to hospital facilities	5.60	1.00	5.30	1.13	2.32	<.021
Opportunity for professional advancement	4.33	1.63	3.83	1.64	2.57	<.011
Teaching medical students, interns or residents	3.68	1.96	3.15	1.87	2.33	<.020
Intellectual stimulation through interaction with colleagues	4.93	1.13	4.53	1.18	2.94	<.004
Working alone	2.76	1.79	3.24	1.87	2.20	<.028
Satisfactory coverage for patients during periods of absence	5.51	1.10	5.12	1.31	2.65	<.009
Personally handling financial aspects of medical practice	4.15	1.89	3.74	1.84	1.80	<.073
Providing some form of patient care outside of the major practice setting (e. g., community clinics, hospitals, etc.)	2.91	1.45	2.50	1.44	2.39	<.018

Responsibility for defining one's role, duties and activities	4.93	1.36	4.58	1.56	1.99	<.048
Personal control of amount of time devoted to patient care	4.85	1.43	4.24	1.65	3.28	<.001
Supervision of subordinates	4.80	1.38	4.47	1.47	1.96	<.051
Expanding one's own knowledge in an area of medicine	4.89	0.99	4.66	1.08	1.91	<.058
Serious financial constraints limiting provision of patient care	2.37	1.53	2.94	1.56	3.07	<.002
Access to new developments in a field of interest or specialization	4.67	1.20	4.32	1.36	2.24	<.026
Opportunity for appreciation and prestige from the lay public	.18	1.61	3.58	1.74	2.98	<.003
Availability of consultation services	5.67	0.72	5.14	1.15	4.57	<.000
Opportunity for appreciation and prestige from colleagues	4.67	1.25	4.10	1.51	3.42	<.001
Working with or under a community board or citizen's group	1.85	1.45	2.20	1.70	1.86	<.065
Taking less vacation and/or free time than one is entitled to take	3.11	1.81	3.65	1.96	2.37	<.019
Maintaining my preferred pace of life	4.53	1.37	3.78	1.62	4.19	<.000
Determining amount of free time and/or vacation time	4.64	1.29	3.88	1.58	4.39	<.000
Sufficient time for family and/or outside activities	4.35	1.42	3.75	1.62	3.33	<.001
Cultural or recreational activities in my geographical area	4.86	1.29	4.30	1.50	3.32	<.001
Availability of desirable public school system	4.96	1.41	4.53	1.61	2.35	<.020
Opportunities for spouse to be employed or pursue preferred activities	4.77	1.56	3.88	1.88	4.20	<.000

Active participation in non-medical community affairs	3.97	1.55	3.44	1.81	2.60	<.010
Opportunity to follow and evaluate patient progress	5.28	1.23	4.94	1.23	2.35	<.019
Cluster 3 Personal control of professional situation	53.03	8.93	45.21	13.94	5.62	<.000
Cluster 4 Medical Innovation	50.10	9.18	45.87	13.38	3.11	<.002
Cluster 5 Personal control of income	55.54	8.33	49.97	13.81	4.11	<.000
Cluster 6 Interaction with the medical community	51.22	9.25	47.13	13.28	3.01	<.003
Cluster 7 Professional prestige	50.19	10.14	44.81	12.81	3.94	<.000

Medical School (Tables 45 and 46)

Medical school faculty appear more satisfied with greater control of their professional lives, intellectual and emotional support from colleagues, and decreased patient interaction. The regression equation shows greater feeling on the Myers-Briggs to increase satisfaction, though the sample contains predominantly thinking types. It would .also appear that other satisfactions to be had in this setting offset amount of income and its control. Typically, medical school faculty earn lower incomes and have less control over it than other practice organizations.

Table 45. Medical School N=66 (S=33; D=33)

	Satisfied		Dissatisfied			
Variable	Mean	SD	Mean	SD	t	p
Items Dr. wants less characteristic	5.84	6.69	11.53	5.56	3.65	<.001
Items Dr. wants more characteristic	12.41	10.68	26.79	9.85	5.64	<.000
Thinking Myers-Briggs	9.02	5.5	12.42	6.14	2.30	<.025
Feeling Myers-Briggs	8.88	6.24	6.03	5.20	2.01	<.048
TF continuous score	92.76	31.93	79.75	28.79	1.73	<.089
Assisting other physicians in performing procedures	3.21	1.69	4.00	1.28	2.14	<.037
Income	2.15	1.54	2.91	1.75	1.84	<.070
Performing therapeutic procedures	2.79	1.78	3.82	1.49	2.55	<.013

Satisfactory coverage for patients during periods of absence	5.00	1.52	4.22	1.83	1.86	<.068
Explaining diagnoses and treatment plans to patients and their families	3.88	1.27	4.42	0.66	2.19	<.034
Access to new developments in a field of interest or specialization	5.48	0.67	5.09	0.86	2.05	<.045
Sharing doubts, frustrations or problems with colleagues	5.13	0.91	4.50	1.52	1.99	<.052
Taking less vacation and/or free time than one is entitled to take	3.63	1.83	4.66	1.60	2.40	<.019
Maintaining my preferred pace of life	4.23	1.59	3.31	1.66	2.24	<.029
Determining amount of free time and/or vacation time	4.29	1.27	3.34	1.60	2.61	<.012
Sufficient time for family and/or outside activities	4.10	1.35	2.81	1.63	3.40	<.001
Cultural or recreational activities in my geographical area	5.26	0.73	3.91	1.65	4.22	<.001
Cluster 3 Personal control of professional situation	48.90	14.60	40.97	13.35	2.30	<.025
Cluster 6 Interaction with the medical community	53.37	7.49	47.64	14.09	2.06	<.044

Table 46. Regression Equation Predicting Satisfaction for Medical School Faculty (N•69)

Variable	Beta Wt.
Cluster 6 - Interaction with medical community	0.4184
Average number of patients seen per week	-0.2780
Thinking - Feeling (Feeling direction)	0.2468
Cluster 1- Medical Innovation	0.2388
Cluster 3 - Personal control of professional situation	0.2185
Judgment - Perception (Judging direction)	-0.1650
Cluster 2 Physician-Teacher	-0.1444
Extraversion - Introversion (Introverted direction)	0.0953
Sensing - Intuition (Intuitive direction)	0.0902
Income .	-0.0838
Cluster 5- Personal control of income	0.0000

TOTAL VARIANCE 0.3705

Institutions (Table 47)

Physicians who have been in their present institutional setting longer are more satisfied than those there a shorter time. In contrast to private practitioners, these physicians appear more satisfied in working with paraprofessionals. The satisfied group has greater interaction with colleagues and is more involved in teaching activities, as well as having more opportunity for innovation and perhaps challenge in their setting. It is interesting, however, that cluster 3-Personal Control of the Professional Situation, does not discriminate satisfied from dissatisfied physicians in institutions. In fact, the t-test indicates that taking less vacation and/or free time . .." is characteristic of the satisfied group, contrary to a11 other analyses of subgroups. It may be the case that this characteristic, when seen within an institutional structure, is associated with increased responsibility and a higher status in the hierarchy of the organization. If this is the case, such individuals may experience greater satisfaction in general than their colleagues who have fewer demands on their time and talents.

Table 47. – Institutions (all hospitals & PHS) N=91 (S=51; D=40)

Variable	Satisfied Mean	SD	Dissatisfied Mean	SD	t	p
Amount of time in present setting	8.27	6.73	6.03	5.58	1.73	<.087
Income	3.58	1.12	2.90	0.91	3.07	<.003
Items rated irrelevant	3.56	5.04	10.67	14.86	2.86	<.006
Items Dr. wants less characteristic	5.23	3.36	7.89	5.82	2.47	<.017
Items Dr. wants more characteristic	12.62	6.08	24.28	12.29	5.43	<.000
Working with paraprofessionals or physician-extenders	4.94	1.3	4.39	1.32	1.9	<.061
Opportunity for affiliation with a medical school	4.51	1.78	3.54	2.16	2.28	<.026
Organizational administration	4.34	0.94	3.56	1.43	2.93	<.005
Dealing with new or unusual patient problems	4.49	1.50	3.89	1.49	1.86	<.086
Delegating certain medical tasks to subordinates	4.67	1.41	3.85	1.77	2.38	<.020
Referring patients to other practitioners or institutions	2.86	1.55	3.39	1.29	1.77	<.081
Presenting cases to some audience	3.31	1.16	2.69	1.24	2.36	<.021

Personal control of amount of time devoted to patient care	4.49	1.50	3.89	1.59	1.79	<.078
Supervision of subordinates	5.51	0.97	4.55	1.58	3.29	<.002
Working with other physicians on some joint task	4.66	1.47	3.90	1.55	2.36	<.021
Access to new developments in a field of interest or specialization	4.80	1.18	4.03	1.57	2.56	<.013
Sharing patient responsibility with other physicians	4.86	1.44	4.00	1.59	2.66	<.010
Isolation from other physicians	1.88	1.42	2.64	1.90	2.09	<.041
Opportunity for prestige and recognition from colleagues	4.65	1.04	3.84	1.50	2.84	<.006
Taking less vacation and/or free time than one is entitled to take	3.69	1.81	2.67	1.74	2.71	<.008
Opportunities for spouse to be employed or pursue preferred activities	5.02	1.34	4.29	1.81	2.07	<.042
Active participation in non-medical community affairs	3.92	1.81	3.18	1.72	1.99	<.050
Cluster 2 Physician Teacher	54.56	8.74	48.54	12.64	2.57	<.012
Cluster 4 Medical Innovation	51.05	9.69	45.21	14.15	2.23	<.029
Cluster 6 Interaction with the medical community	5.12	10.10	45.01	13.64	2.41	<.018
Cluster 7 Professional prestige	51.02	7.91	45.26	13.86	2.31	<.025

The remaining analyses of practice organizations examine specific groups in order to describe more precisely the factors contributing to satisfaction in relation to -these settings.

Solo Private Practice (Table 48 and 49)

Solo private practitioners appear to gain satisfaction both from greater control over their income, as well as independence in the conduct of their practices. The occurrence of items dealing with counseling and treatment of emotional problems may be influenced by the large number of psychiatrists in private practice settings in this sample. It is notable that extent of personal patient involvement (cluster 1) is a source of satisfaction for solo private practitioners, even though the regression equation indicates that seeing fewer patients is related to increased satisfaction. Those with greater extraversion, intuition, feeling and judgment appear more satisfied in this sample. For all type preferences, except judgment-perception, the opposite types predominate in the sample.

Table 48. Solo Private Practice N=58 (S=30; D=28)

Variable	Satisfied		Dissatisfied		t	p
	Mean	SD	Mean	SD		
Items Dr. wants less characteristic	4.50	2.91	11.25	7.36	4.24	<.000
Items Dr. wants more characteristic	12.52	5.93	23.07	11.88	4.22	<.000
Dealing with ethical or moral issues in the practice of medicine	4.97	1.16	4.00	1.54	2.65	<.011
Personal control of amount of earnings	5.10	1.24	4.36	1.62	1.95	<.056
Availability of hospital facilities	5.67	1.06	5.00	1.44	2.00	<.052
Satisfactory coverage for patients during periods of absence	5.27	1.48	4.41	1.47	2.19	<.033
Personally handling financial aspects of medical practice	5.23	1.25	3.74	1.97	3.37	<.002
Responsibility for defining one's role, duties and activities	5.55	0.91	4.54	1.82	2.66	<.011
Dealing with patients' emotional difficulties	5.30	1.09	4.54	1.62	2.09	<.042
Sharing doubts, frustrations or problems with colleagues	4.17	1.56	3.52	1.12	1.8	<.087
Advising or counseling patients and/or their families	5.57	1.07	4.96	1.06	2.14	<.037
Availability of consultation services	5.93	0.25	4.85	1.29	4.28	<.000
Cultural or recreational activities in my geographical area	4.83	1.15	3.73	1.76	2.74	<.009
Availability of desirable public school system	5.40	1.13	3.96	1.76	3.58	<.001
Opportunities for spouse to be employed or pursue preferred activities	5.21	1.42	3.38	2.02	3.82	<.000

Active participation in non-medical community affairs	3.72	1.71	2.74	1.68	2.17	<.034
Cluster 1 Personal patient involvement	56.69	6.46	53.67	6.27	1.81	<.076
Cluster 3 Personal control of professional situation	52.72	8.60	46.63	15.26	1.85	<.071
Cluster 5 Personal control of income	60.63	6.13	54.31	7.80	3.41	<.001

Table 49. Regression Equation Predicting Satisfaction for Solo Private Practice (N-60)

Variable	Beta Wt.
Cluster 6 - Interaction with medical community	0.4506
Cluster 7 - Professional prestige	-0.4393
Cluster 5 - Personal control of income	0.4202
Cluster 3 - Personal control of professional situation	0.3423
Income	0.3327
Cluster 2 – Physician -Teache	0.2533
Thinking - Feel1ng (Feeling direction)	0.2151
Extraversion - Introversion (Extraverted direction)	-0.2031
Judgment - Perception (Judgment direction.)	-0.1121
Average number patients seen per week	-0.0885
Cluster 4 - Medical innovation	-0.0881
Cluster 1 - Personal patient involvement	0.0648
Sensing - Intuition (Intuitive direction)	0.0396
Year of graduation from medical school	-0.0376
TOTAL VARIANCE	0.4989

Partnerships (Tables 50 and 51)

Amount of Personal Patient Involvement does not discriminate satisfied .from dissatisfied groups, though it appears in the regression equation as predictive of satisfaction. These physicians appear more satisfied when they have less interaction with their colleagues and other medical facilities and through personal control of income (cluster 5) increases satisfaction, those with lower income are more likely to be satisfied.

As observed before, there would appear two factors intervening in the income-satisfaction relationship for this group. In terms of personality type, physicians in partnerships appear more satisfied with greater extraversion, intuition, thinking and judgment. This does. not deviate markedly from the type distribution for this sample, except for extraversion - introversion where the sample is largely made up of introverted types.

Table 50. Partnership N=65 (S=34; D=31)

	Satisfied		Dissatisfied			
Variable	Mean	SD	Mean	SD	t	p
Pre-college community size	2.91	1.46	2.00	1.18	2.77	<.007
Items Dr. wants less characteristic	5.71	3.90	10.10	6.84	3.10	<.003
Items Dr. wants more characteristic	12.31	6.48	23.39	11.25	4.77	<.000
Introversion on Myers-Briggs	14.15	6.15	11.45	6.46	1.72	<.091
Dealing with emergency medical problems	5.00	0.99	4.46	1.35	1.75	<.086
Personal control of amount of earnings	4.62	1.48	3.93	1.54	1.79	<.079
Opportunity for affiliation with a medical school	2.97	2.14	3.89	2.01	1.74	<.088
Working alone	2.30	1.53	3.89	1.57	3.98	<.000
Performing diagnostic procedures	3.88	1.67	3.07	1.94	1.77	<.083
Responsibility for defining one's role, duties and activities	5.16	1.04	4.30	1.54	2.47	<.017
Personal control of amount of time devoted to patient care	4.94	1.14	4.25	1.46	2.03	<.048
Supervision of subordinates	5.09	1.00	4.07	1.14	3.21	<.002
Trying out new ideas	4.62	0.89	3.86	1.32	2.59	<.013
Expanding one's own knowledge in an area of medicine	5.03	0.97	4.54	0.96	2.01	<.050
Serious financial constraints limiting provision of patient care	2.33	1.36	3.36	1.66	2.60	<.012
Opportunity for appreciation and prestige from						

the lay public	4.97	1.06	4.04	1.71	2.52	<.015
Availability of consultation services	5.79	0.48	5.46	0.79	1.93	<.060
Opportunity for prestige and recognition from colleagues	4.85	0.89	4.07	1.52	2.36	<.023
Taking less vacation and/or free time than one is entitled to take	2.97	1.70	4.11	1.63	2.65	<.011
Cluster 3 Personal control of professional situation	52.58	8.83	45.02	17.35	2,18	<.034
Cluster 4 Medical innovation	51.08	8.48	41.93	16.25	2.81	<.007

Table 51. Regression Equation Predicting Satisfaction for Partnerships (N=67)

Variable	Beta Wt.
Cluster 6 -- Interaction with medical community	-0.3699
Cluster 4 - Medical innovation	0.3460
Cluster 5 - Personal control of income	0.2759
Cluster 7 Professional prestige	0.2613
Income	-0.2537
Pre-college community size (larger communities)	0.2005
Cluster 2- Physician-Teacher	-0.1874
Community size (larger communities)	0.1749
Extraversion - Introversion (extraverted direction)	-0.1666
Judgment - Perception (judgmental direction)	-0.1375
Cluster 1 - Personal patient involvement	0.1294
Year of graduation from medical school	0.1289
Thinking - Feeling (Thinking direction)	-0.1239
Cluster 3 - Personal control of professional situation	-0.1152
Sensing - Intuition (Intuitive direction)	0.0539
TOTAL VARIANCE	0.4533

Small Groups (Tables 52 and 53)

Physicians in small groups differ in several ways from those in partnerships, though they are similar in the negative relationship of interaction with the medical community and satisfaction, as well as the importance of controlling income and professional prestige. Personal Control of the Professional Situation is of most importance for this group, where it appears negatively related to satisfaction for physicians in partnerships. Medical innovation shows a negative relationship for physicians in small groups, and a positive one for partnerships. It would appear therefore, that the work situation of several physicians who practice together is quite different from one where two physicians are partners. This is further suggested by the indication that greater introversion is associated with satisfaction for small groups where greater extraversion leads to satisfaction for partnerships.

Table 52. Small Group, Same Specialty N=98 (S=51; D=47)

Variable	Satisfied Mean	SD	Dissatisfied Mean	SD	t	p
Items Dr. wants less characteristic	6.04	4.23	12.47	6.08	5.72	<.000
Items Dr. wants more characteristic	12.17	5.72	28.09	10.29	9.24	<.000
Working with paraprofessionals or physician extenders	3.96	1.53	4.66	1.26	2.24	<.028
Maintaining a fairly consistent and predictable patient-scheduling system	4.56	1.54	3.63	1.68	2.66	<.010
Personal control of amount of earnings	4.61	1.33	3.42	1.70	3.77	<.000
Opportunity for professional advancement	4.16	1.73	3.49	1.70	1.90	<.060
Teaching medical students, interns or residents	3.78	1.95	2.96	1.88	2.12	<.037
Intellectual stimulation through interaction with colleagues	5.04	0.98	4.53	1.22	2.22	<.029
Supervision and/or teaching medical students or medical personnel	3.94	1.05	3.50	1.28	1.85	<.068
Providing some form of patient care outside of the major practice setting	2.92	1.41	2.33	1.38	2.10	<.039
Personal control of amount of time devoted to patient care	4.82	1.45	3.73	1.72	3.31	<.001
Sharing patient responsibility with other physicians	4.90	1.27	4.2	1.60	2.34	<.021
Opportunity for prestige and recognition from colleagues	4.49	1.36	3.96	1.57	1.77	<.080
Maintaining my preferred pace of life	4.45	1.39	3.40	1.57	3.45	<.001
Determining amount of free time and/or vacation time	4.57	1.38	3.58	1.50	3.36	<.001
Sufficient time for family and/or outside	4.45	1.49	3.58	1.55	2.81	<.006

activities						
Cultural or recreational activities in my geographical area	5.12	1.23	4.33	1.37	2.94	<.004
Opportunities for spouse to be employed or pursue preferred activities	4.67	1.62	4.00	1.80	1.86	<.086
Opportunity to follow and evaluate patient progress	5.12	1.29	4.53	1.36	2.15	<.034
Cluster 2 Physician-Teacher	49.60	8.29	46.39	9.10	1.82	<.072
Cluster 3 Personal control of professional situation	53.53	8.95	43.58	13.51	4.26	<.000
Cluster 5 Personal control of income	56.16	6.98	49.37	13.63	3.06	<.003
Cluster 6 Interaction with the medical community	52.10	8.89	47.56	13.55	1.94	<.056
Cluster 7 Professional prestige	49.02	10.15	42.94	12.45	2.64	<.010

Table 53. Regression Equation Predicting Satisfaction for Small Groups (same or mixed specialties) (N=105)

Variable	Beta Wt.
Cluster 3 - Personal control of professional situation	0.4244
Cluster 4 - Medical Innovation	-0.1679
Cluster 7 - Professional prestige	0.1549
Cluster 5 - Personal control of income	0.1466
Pre-college community size (Larger communities)	0.1246
Cluster 1 - Personal patient involvement	0.1184
Cluster 2 - Physician-.Teacher	0.0838
Year of graduation from medical school	0.0732
Extraversion - Introversion (introverted direction)	0.0409
Income	0.0362
Cluster 6 - Interaction with medical community	-0.0359
Average number of patients seen per week	-0.0233
Sensing - Intuition (Intuitive direction)	0.0219
TOTAL VARIANCE	0.3236

Large Group Practice (Table 54)

The sample for this regression equation included groups of seven or more physicians, including hospital based groups. Satisfaction for these physicians is increased by increased income, more opportunity for innovation and the perhaps related variable of seeing fewer patients, though satisfaction is increased by greater involvement with patients. Practicing and interacting with the medical community are negatively associated with satisfaction for large group physicians. Those who are more recent graduates of medical school, and therefore younger, appear more satisfied than their older colleagues in this setting. In terms of personality type, greater introversion, sensing, feeling and perception tend to increase satisfaction.

Table 54. Regression Equation Predicting Satisfaction for Large Group Practice (N=53)

Variable	Beta Wt.
Income	0.4200
Cluster 4 - Medical innovation	0.2981
Average number of patients seen per week	-0.2334
Thinking - Feeling (Feeling direction)	0.2206
Cluster 3 - Personal control of professional situation	0.1742
Cluster 1 - Personal patient involvement	0.1624
Sensing - Intuition (Sensing direction)	-0.1583
Cluster 2 - Physician-teacher	-0.1522
Cluster 6 - Interaction with medical community	-0.1316
Cluster 7 - Professional prestige	0.1124
Pre-college community size (Larger communities)	0.0921
Judgment- Perception (Perceptive direction	0.0634
Year of graduation from medical school	0.0491
Cluster 5 - Personal control of income	-0.0348
Extraversion - Introversion (Introverted direction)	0.0273
TOTAL VARIANCE	0.3905

Non-Government Hospitals (Table 55)

Sources of satisfaction for these physicians include practicing in larger communities, seeing a greater number of patients., not being involved in medical innovation and teaching and less control of the professional situation. As previously observed, the latter negative association with satisfaction is probably explained via some set of satisfiers inherent in certain settings which offsets the usually undesirable lack of control of the professional situation. Greater introversion, sensing and perception also tend to increase satisfaction. The sample is largely introverted and judgmental in the distribution of the types.

Table 55. Regression Equation Predicting Satisfaction for Physicians in Non-government Hospitals (N=25)

Variable	Beta Wt.
Judgment - Perception (Perceptive direction)·	2.4926
Sensing - Intuition (Sensing direction)	-2.3476
Community size (larger communities)	0.7895
Average number of patients seen per week	0.7748
Extraversion - Introversion (Introverted direction)	0.6561
Cluster 3 - Personal control of professional situation	-0.5727
Cluster 2 – Physician teacher	-0.2298
Pre-college community size (smaller communities)	-0.1524
Cluster 4- Medical innovation	-0.0455
TOTAL VARIANCE	0.9931

Government Hospital and the Public Health Service (Table 56)

This sample includes city. county and state hospitals, military hospitals, the VA and Public Health Service hospitals. Sample sizes for these individual settings were too small for separate analysis. As compared to non-government hospitals, physicians in this setting have increased satisfaction through teaching, medical innovation and seeing fewer patients. They also tend to come from larger communities and like most other groups studied, their satisfaction is increased with greater control of the professional situation and increased income.

Table 56. - Regression Equation Predicting Satisfaction for Physicians in Government Hospitals and Public Health Service (N=56)

Variable	Beta Wt.
Cluster 1 - Professional prestige	-0.6003
Cluster 2 - Physician-Teacher	0.4595
Cluster 6 - Interaction with medical community	0.4387
Cluster 4 - Medical innovation	0.2372
Average number of patients seen per week	-0.1975
Year of graduation from medical school	-0.1518
Judgment - Perception (Judgmental direction)	-0.1175
Cluster 5 - Personal control of income	-0.1020
Community size (larger communities)	0.8876
Pre-college community size (larger communities)	0.0858
Cluster 1 - Personal patient· involvement	-0.0762

Income	0.0749
Cluster 3 - Personal control of professional situation	0.0721
Thinking - Feeling (Thinking direction)	-0.0148
TOTAL VARIANCE	0.4335

Summary of satisfaction for practice organizations

In examining variables that are of importance for 3 or more of the six practice organizations described, the following occur:

>Cluster 3- Personal Control of the Professional Situation (5 groups)
>Personal control of amount of time devoted to patient care (4 groups)
>Supervision of subordinates (4 groups)
>Personal control of amount of earnings (4 groups)
>Opportunity for prestige and recognition from colleagues (4 groups)
>Taking less vacation or free time than one is entitled to take (4 groups)
>Cultural or recreational activities in my geographic area (4 groups)
>Opportunities for spouse to be employed or pursue preferred activities (4 groups)
>Cluster 5- Personal Control of Income (4 groups)
>Cluster 6- Interaction with the medical community (4 groups)
>Responsibility for defining one's role, duties and activities (3 groups)
>Access to new developments in a field of interest of specialization (3 groups)
>Working alone (3 groups)
>Satisfactory coverage for patients during periods of absence (3 groups)
>Accessibility of consultation services (3 groups)
>Maintaining my preferred pace of life (3 groups)
>Determining amount of free time or vacation time (3 groups)
>Sufficient time for family or outside activities (3 groups)
>Cluster 4- Medical Innovation (3 groups)

Although there are evident idiosyncrasies characteristic of sources of satisfaction within certain practice organizations,it appears that the same kinds of factors are important discriminators no matter what subgroup is being considered. Larger samples in some of the distinct practice organizations such as military hospitals, would permit a more precise understanding of the characteristics which increase and decrease satisfaction for physicians. The present data, however, provide some insight into both general and specific differentiators of satisfaction for these practice organizations.

Discussion

Several outcomes of this study of physician satisfaction are noteworthy. In general, the image of the satisfied physician in looking at results for the total sample, is that he (she) enjoys having challenging work, collaborating and/or having available the expertise of other health professionals as opposed to working alone, having a satisfactory personal life for spouse and family, sharing acquired knowledge through supervision and teaching, controlling the amount of earnings and earning a higher income.

It is interesting that though in many cases increased income is a source of satisfaction, in others it appears to be offset by other negative features such that it appears that a physician may be satisfied with less money if other more important sources of satisfaction are available. This observation has implications for certain kinds of settings which are typically characterized by lower income. It suggests both that increasing physician income in these settings may be an insufficient motivator for recruitment and retention, and also points to the necessity for altering the characteristics of these settings to provide a greater opportunity for attempting to recruit and retain· physicians in government hospitals, it would seem worthwhile to attempt to maximize the opportunities for teaching, building positive attributes associated with. physician satisfaction in these settings. Similar clues are provided for other practice organizations as well as particular specialties. Unfortunately, the opportunity to observe the interaction of specialty and practice organization in relation to differential satisfaction was not possible due to the small samples available in these more specific subgroups. Theoretically with larger samples, it would be possible to delineate the important sources of' satisfaction for such groups as radiologic therapists in VA hospitals. Using such- information based upon empirical evidence would maximize the possibilities of creating. effective recruitment and retention policies for under-served settings and specialties.

The observation that for most physicians, working alone and in isolation from others is a source of dissatisfaction, is consonant with the observed dispreferences of current medical students and young physicians for solo private practice. It also provides an additional rationale for encouraging .the team approach to the delivery of medical care, especially in rural under-served settings which cannot provide the intellectual stimulation or consultation services available in urban areas.

Also of interest is the confirmation in these results of the belief that spouse's needs are important to physician motivation and satisfaction. This is true for the sample as a whole as well as a large number of subgroups. It implies that the career decisions of physicians may be influenced by opportunities available for the spouse and that attention to spouse characteristics should be an important consideration in planning and implementing innovative health care delivery systems in remote areas.

The frequently observed relationship between increased satisfaction and higher scores on personality type preferences which are infrequent in particular samples, suggests that perhaps more extreme type preferences in an individual are a liability with respect to satisfaction. It would appear that, for example, the intuitive psychiatrist who has potentially available to him at· least some preferences or abilities for sensing activities. is more likely to be satisfied than his colleague who is more one-sided in his preference for intuition. And the introverted anesthesiologist who has more "available" extraversion, may fare better than the extremely introverted anesthesiologist. These clues to type preference functioning may prove to be important in future investigations of type relationships. To date data relating type preferences to differential satisfaction have not been available for study. It would seem worthwhile to pursue further collection of similar information for other groups of individuals in order to further elucidate these more subtle relationships between type preference and career satisfaction.

Finally, detailed information on sources of career satisfaction for specialties and practice organizations is potentially useful for counseling and advising medical students and young physicians who are in the process of making important career decisions. These data, which take into account the personality type preferences, career characteristics, and their interaction, can provide a more objective basis for career choices than is currently available in the field of medicine. The availability of such information may permit the young physician to correct possible misconceptions about a particular specialty or practice organization by providing a more accurate picture of what is is like to practice a specialty. This should temper what may be an inaccurate image of practice which is based upon experience limited to hospital settings and medical school physicians.

Using such information, the young physician may discover potentially satisfying practice situations of which he may have been unaware, as well as enabling him to reject as potentially unsatisfying, practice styles which he may have seriously considered. The end result of this kind of use of the information should be to maximize the "accuracy" of career choice decisions at an earlier stage of career development. This would eliminate much trial and error inherent in "trying out" careers, which would hopefully increase both career satisfaction for physicians as well as continuity and quality of care for consumers of medical care.

Further, government agencies and others concerned with recruiting physicians for under-served specialties and settings, can use this information to orient their search for candidates to the most appropriate kinds of aspiring physicians. This should serve to reduce turnover currently characteristic in such agencies as the National Health Service Corps, by enabling recruitment of physicians who would be more likely to remain in the corps. In addition, the present data provide specific suggestions with regard to the kinds of changes in practice characteristics which may be necessary in order to attract young physicians to such settings and retain them by satisfying their career needs.

Addendum: VA Physicians

Of the 477 respondents to the larger study, fifteen were full-time V.A. physicians and twelve were associated with the V.A. on a part-time basis. Although it would be desirable to have a larger representation of V.A. physicians, comparisons with other samples of institutionally affiliated physicians suggest that these respondents are representative of institutional physicians in terms of patient attributes, personality styles and common practice characteristics. We may thus evaluate differences between V.A. physicians and a cross-section of physicians in other practice organizations as fairly reliable indicies of differentiating characteristics which may be observed in any future study of larger samples of V.A. Physicians.

The list of physicians from which samples were drawn for the larger study was obtained through the American Medical Association and initial designations of sampling criteria were based upon A.M.A. information. These criteria were such that respondents represented five geographic areas of the country, five sizes of community, fourteen specialty areas, and eleven practice organizations. Final classification on these variables was made on the basis of information provided by physicians in responding to the Physician Work Setting Instrument (PWSI), the major data collection instrument of the project. All physicians who were selected had received the M.D. degree between 1945 and 1965. The sample of V.A. physicians did not differ significantly from the remainder of the sample in their representation of different areas of the country or in the size of the communities in which they practiced. The medical specialties included in the group were: internal medicine, psychiatry, general surgery, orthopedic surgery, pathology and radiology.

Data Analysis Techniques

The combined sample of full- and part-time V.A. physicians (N=27) was compared with the remaining physicians in the larger study (N=450). Comparisons were made on all variables reflecting practice characteristics, including scores on the seven clusters as well as scores on individual activity and characteristic items; on an overall score of satisfaction with their work situation (the sum of the items the physician indicated he would like "to remain the same" in his practice); and on scores on Myers- Briggs Type Indicator preferences. A second analysis compared these same variables for full-time V.A. physicians versus part-time affiliates. All comparisons used the t-test for the significance of differences between means.

A further analysis sought to delineate the factors associated with satisfaction for the two groups. The statistical technique called multiple regression was used to evaluate the relative contributions of variables to the prediction of overall satisfaction as measured by the previously described summative score. This technique produces a linear combination of independent variables (those hypothesized to contribute to satisfaction) which are weighted so as to maximize the correlation with the dependent variable (satisfaction), while taking into account the intercorrelations among the independent variables. The magnitude of weights assigned to the independent variables in the resulting prediction equation (the Beta weights) reflects the strength and direction of the direct relationship between the independent variables and the dependent variable. Interest was in the kinds of factors associated with satisfaction for V.A. Physicians.

Results

Differences Between Total V.A. Sample and Non-V.A. Physicians

Table 57 shows the means, standard deviations, t values and significance levels for comparisons of the combined sample of V.A. full-time and part-time physicians- and all non-V.A. affiliated physicians. As can be seen, V.A. physicians participated frequently in patient-related activities (e. g. performing therapeutic procedures; explaining diagnoses; dealing with emotional problems). However, they more often engage in teaching and supervisory activities and tend to be affiliated with medical schools. As expected, they have less control over their incomes and indeed earn less than other physicians, as well as engaging more frequently in organizational administration. It might be expected that working in an institutional setting would permit greater ability to control "life style" factors. However, items reflecting such factors were not significantly different for the two groups. Overall satisfaction, which was also hypothesized to be lower for V.A. physicians , is not significantly different for this combined sample. Analysis of full- versus part-time V.A. physicians, however, is interesting in pinpointing some of these kinds of differences.

Table 57. Means, standard deviations and comparisons between VA and Non-VA Physicians.

Variables	VA		Non-VA			
	Mean	SD	Mean	SD	t	p
Average Number of Patients Seen Per week	65.37	68.80	102.70	84.61	1.89	<.05
Number of Regular Settings	1.68	0.95	1.16	0.45	4.23	<.005
Income of Physician (1= less than 20,000; 5 = 50,000 +)	3.28	0.61	4.04	1.1	3.4	<.005
Cluster 1 - Personal Patient Involvement*	44.13	13.30	50.11	10.24	2.84	<.005
Cluster 2 - Physician Teacher	58.37	5.63	49.29	10.51	4.36	<.005
Cluster 5 - Personal Control of Income	40.90	7.67	49.64	11.86	3.71	<.005
Dealing with Ethical or Moral Issues in the Practice of Medicine (item)**	3.69	1.89	4.12	1.52	1.38	<.10
Working with Paraprofessionals or Physician Extenders (item)	4.7	1.36	4.17	1.56	1.58	<.10
Dealing with Emergency Medical Problems (item)	3.80	1.80	4.18	1.52	3.10	<.005
Personal Control of Amount of Earnings (item)	1.79	1.41	3.58	1.85	4.65	<.005
Opportunity for Affiliation with a Medical School (item)**	5.23	1.63	3.81	2.09	3.41	<.005
Teaching Medical Students, Interns or Residents (item)	5.23	1.24	3.86	1.96	3.53	<.005
Organizational Administration (item)	4.15	0.97	3.71	1.10	2.01	<.025
Performing Therapeutic Procedures (item)	3.00	1.93	3.65	1.65	1.87	<.05
Dealing with New or Unusual Patient Problems (item)	4.19	1.77	4.55	1.21	1.43	<.10
Personally Handling Financial Aspects of Medical Care (item)	1.8	1.58	3.35	2	3.79	<.005
Referring Patients to other Practitioners	3.12	1.54	3.56	1.35	1.56	<.10

(item)						
Providing Some Form of Patient Care Outside of the Regular Setting	1.96	1.46	2.65	1.46	2.29	<.025
Presenting Cases to Some Audience (item)	3.54	0.88	2.84	1.15	2.92	<.005
Explaining Diagnoses and Treatment Plans to Patients and/or their Families (item)	3.67	1.58	4.4	1.16	2.96	<.005
Expanding one's own knowledge in an area of medicine (item)	4.58	1.33	4.88	1.03	1.42	<.10
Dealing with patients' emotional problems (item)	3.40	2.04	4.15	1.70	2.12	<.025
Access to new developments in a field of interest or specialization (item)	4.31	1.57	4.65	1.25	1.33	<.10
Advising or counseling patients and/or their families (item)	3.52	1.9	4.27	1.79	2.01	<.025
Opportunity for appreciation and prestige from the lay public (item)	2.77	1.7	3.77	1.67	2.96	<.005
Accessibility of consultation services (item)	5.11	1.34	5.40	1.00	1.38	<.10
Direct patient contact (item)	4.15	2.13	5.07	1.55	2.84	<.005
Determining amount of free time and/or vacation time (item)	3.39	1.84	4.18	1.5	2.58	<.005
Opportunity to follow and evaluate patient progress (item)	4.54	1.55	4.96	1.37	1.51	<.10
Sum of items judged irrelevant (to satisfaction)	7.50	11.87	3.96	8.65	1.98	<.025
Sensing-Intuition on the Myers-Briggs (High score = Intuitive)	104.68	26.31	93.65	33.04	1.64	<.10
Medical record time keeping (item)	4.29	1.33	4.44	1.11	0.65	ns
Trying Out New Ideas (item}	4.39	1.20	4.44	1.22	0.23	ns
Sharing patient responsibility with other physicians (item)	4.73	1.49	4.57	1.45	0.55	ns

Maintaining a fairly consistent and predictable patient scheduling system	4.21	2.09	4.45	1.63	0.65	ns
Opportunity for professional advancement	4.16	1.55	4.26	1.61	0.29	ns
Performing habitual or non-varying medical activities (item)	3.84	1.65	3.83	1.53	0.04	ns
Taking less vacation and/or free time than one is entitled to take	3.77	1.97	3.44	1.87	0.86	ns
Maintaining my preferred "pace of life" (item)	3.96	1.51	4.15	1.54	0.62	ns
Sufficient time for family and/or outside activities (item)	4.42	1.42	4.03	1.6	1.23	ns
Overall satisfaction (sum of items physicians would like to remain "the same")	32.17	14.01	30.24	15.23	0.61	ns

* Cluster scores are standardized so that the mean for the entire sample of 477 physicians = 50 and the standard deviation = 10. Scores of approximately 45 may be considered moderately low; scores of approximately 55, moderately high.

** A six-point scale of "characteristicness" was used, ranging from I = very uncharacteristic to 6 = very characteristic.

Differences Between Full-time and Part-time V.A. Physicians

Table 58 provides the same kind of information as Table 57 for the comparison of the two sub-samples of V.A. physicians. Some striking differences are evident between these two subgroups, notably the difference in overall satisfaction. Full-time V.A. physicians are considerably less satisfied than their part-time colleagues, in spite of the fact that they have remained in the V.A. significantly longer and are an average of seven years older. In addition, full-time physicians do less teaching and are less often affiliated with a medical school, are less professionally ambitious and see less opportunity for professional advancement. In terms of patient care activities, the full-time physicians are less focused on special interest areas, more often work alone, more often perform habitual medical tasks and less often deal with unusual medical care problems. However, full-time people, probably by virtue of occupying only a single work setting, read journals more often, expand their own knowledge in medicine and have better control over their free time and activities outside of medicine in the form of greater personal control: of the professional situation. This combination of work setting attributes, however, appears to be less satisfying than the opposite characteristics which are associated with part-time V.A. affiliation. Because of the striking differences between the full-time and part-time V.A. physicians, regression equations were generated separately for the two sub-groups in order to compare their sources of satisfaction.

Table 58. List of Variables discriminating full-time and part-time VA Physicians

Variables	Full-time Mean	SD	Part-time Mean	SD	t	p
Length of Time in Present Setting (Years)	10.20	6.96	5.36	3.78	2.08	0.00
Income (l=less than 20,000;5=50,000 +)	3.00	0.38	3.70	0.68	3.33	0.00
Year of graduation from medical school	54.80	6.68	58.45	5.11	1.52	0.00
Age (Years)	47.31	8.81	40.29	4.31	1.97	0.00
Cluster 2 - Physician Teacher*	56.70	6.16	60.64	4.04	1.84	0.00
Cluster 3 - Personal Control of Professional Situation	51.03	8.45	45.98	9.55	1.42	0.00
Cluster 7 - Professional Ambition	46.92	9.53	54.45	8.13	2.11	0.00
Reading journals and medical books (item)••	4.67	0.49	4.09	0.70	2.47	0.00
Opportunity for affiliation with a medical school (item)	4.80	2.04	0.00	0.40	1.62	0.00
Focus on a special interest area within a specialty (item)	3.67	1.50	5.18	0.98	2.92	0.00
Opportunity for professional advancement (item)	3.67	1.63	4.90	1.10	2.09	0.00
Teaching medical students, interns or residents (item)	4.80	1.47	5.82	0.40	2.22	0.00
Performing habitual or non-varying medical tasks (item)	4.29	1.68	3.27	1.49	1.57	0.00
Working alone (little assistance from other medical personnel) (item)	3.20	1.86	1.55	1.21	2.57	0.00
Dealing with new or unusual patient problems (items)	3.73	1.79	4.82	1.60	1.59	0.00
Personally handling financial aspects of medical practice (item)	1.29	1.07	2.45	1.92	1.94	0.00
Personal control of amount of time devoted	3.79	1.85	4.91	0.94	1.83	0.00

to patient care (item)						
Expanding one's own knowledge in an area of medicine (item)	4.87	1.36	4.18	1.25	1.31	0.00
Opportunity for appreciation and prestige from the lay public (item)	2.40	1.68	3.27	1.68	1.31	0.00
Taking less vacation and/or free time than one is entitled to take (item)	3.00	2.03	4.82	1.33	2.58	0.00
Maintaining my preferred pace of life (item)	4.40	1.45	3.36	1.43	1.81	0.00
Sufficient time for family and/or outside activities (item)	4.87	1.45	3.82	1.17	1.96	0.00

Differences in Sources of Satisfaction for Full-time and Part-time V.A. Physicians

The variables included as predictors in the multiple regression analysis were selected on the basis of judgments made as to their probable influence on satisfaction. The overall measure of satisfaction previously described was the dependent variable. Multiple regression technique allows the determination of the per cent of the variation in the dependent variable which is attributable to variation in the set of independent predictor variables included in the regression equation. Accounting for 100% of the variance would represent perfect prediction, i. e. knowledge of scores on the variables in the equation would allow us to perfectly predict scores on satisfaction. Accounting for 50% of the variance means that half of the variation in satisfaction is attributable to the variation in the variables in the prediction equation. The remaining 50% is attributable to some combination of measurement error and other variables not included in the equation.

More often than not, the range of variance accounted for in the social sciences is less than 50%, with 30 to 40% considered quite good. The accuracy of prediction found here, (91% of the variance for full-time and 93% of the variance for part-time), is therefore high, especially in light of the small numbers of variables required to achieve these levels of prediction.

Table 59 shows the variables included in the regression equations for the two groups. In all, seven variables were selected for possible inclusion in both equations. Of these, one did not account for sufficient variance for inclusion in either equation. This was Cluster 1 - Personal Patient Involvement.

Table 59. Regression Equations Predicting Satisfaction for Full-Time and Part-Time VA Physicians.

Variable	Beta Weight	
	Full Time VA	Part-time VA
Cluster 2 - Physician Teacher	1.92**	

Cluster 3 - Personal Control of Professional Situation		2.17*
Cluster 7 - Professional Ambition	0.02*	-3.10***
Average Number Patients Seen Per Week	-1.74**	
Physician Income	0.21*	2.47*
Sensing-Intuition on the Myers-Briggs	-0.88#	2.68##
Total Variance Accounted for	91.00%	93.00%

*High score = greater satisfaction
** Low score = greater satisfaction
\# Sensing = greater satisfaction
\#\# Intuition = greater satisfaction

Comparison of the regression equations indicates quite different patterns of satisfaction for the two kinds of V.A. physicians. In light of the low income characteristic of V.A. physicians in comparison to physicians in other work settings, it is not surprising that for both groups higher income is associated with increased satisfaction. However, this appears to be the only similarity between the two groups.

For full-time V.A. physicians increased satisfaction is associated with increased teaching activity and professional ambition and dealing with fewer patients. In addition, those full-time physicians who have higher Sensing scores on the Myers-Briggs are more satisfied than those with higher scores on Intuition. This appears to correspond to the characteristics of full-time V.A. employment as described in Table 4. A preference for Sensing is associated with a preference for dealing with more routine, present-oriented activities and less enjoyment of complex problem-solving situations. Physicians with higher Intuition scores would likely be dissatisfied in a highly structured organizational setting which provides decreased opportunity for innovation and independent professional pursuits. If the characterization of full-time V.A. employment obtained in this study is, in general, accurate, it seems appropriate that physicians who enjoy "Sensing" situations would be more satisfied than their more intuitive colleagues.

Part-time V.A. physicians, however, who frequently use their non-V.A. time in medical schools and similar educational settings, are more satisfied if they have higher scores on Intuition. Working in two settings presumably permits greater opportunity for engaging in a more complex array of activities. These physicians are similar in this characteristic to full-time medical school faculty, who are, in general, higher in Intuition than Sensing (Myers and Davis, 1965). Part-time V.A. physicians also derive greater satisfaction if they have greater personal control of their professional situations. In the larger study, high scores on this factor were always associated with increased satisfaction and low scores invariably reflected dissatisfaction. Full-time physicians apparently do not vary sufficiently on this factor for it to be of any consequence. They all have a high level of control in this area. Similarly, the part-time practitioners are all high in teaching activities so that this factor appears irrelevant to satisfaction for them. However, it appears that decreased focus on variables reflecting professional ambition is associated with increased satisfaction for part-time physicians. It appears likely that though there may be opportunity for professional advancement in one or both of the regular work settings of part-time physicians, these opportunities may not be open to them because of their part-time status. Thus, they may experience greater dissatisfaction in comparing themselves to full-time colleagues for whom the items included in this cluster are more accessible. By contrast, part-time physicians who may see little opportunity for advancement for themselves or their full-time colleagues, may not focus on these factors and would thus appear more satisfied.

It should be emphasized, however, that although these results, "make sense," sample sizes available for these regression equations make the results quite tentative. They are suggestive of hypotheses that must be tested on much larger samples of physicians.

Discussion

The results of this study have several implications with regard to the attraction and retention of physicians in V.A. hospitals. The fact that full-time V.A. physicians are more dissatisfied with their total situation than their part-time colleagues suggests that the characteristics of full-time V.A. employment are inherently dissatisfying to physicians in general. In addition, the kinds of personal and work setting attributes associated with increased satisfaction in a full-time V.A. setting suggest that a very limited segment of the physician population would be satisfied in V.A. hospitals. Further, since Sensing on the Myers-Briggs was associated with increased satisfaction, it is well to point out that for a combined sample of 2000 medical students from a cross-section of medical schools there are nearly twice as many Intuitive as Sensing types [79]. Thus the available pool of physicians who may find career satisfaction in the V.A. is much more limited than it would be if this work setting included potential satisfaction for intuitive physicians as well.

Though it seems clear that increasing V.A. salaries would probably increase physician satisfaction, it appears unlikely that this in itself will make full-time V.A. employment more attractive to physicians. Rather, the present data suggest that in order to increase the attractiveness of the V.A. and its ability to retain highly motivated and skilled physicians, the opportunities available in the setting require innovative alteration. Increasing the opportunity for physicians to engage in more novel medical care delivery, perhaps expanded availability of research opportunities, and less focus on routine patient care and administrative work would broaden the spectrum of physicians who might obtain career satisfaction in the V.A.

It may also become apparent when larger samples are studied that work setting characteristics and satisfactions differ among medical specialties within the V.A. Regression equations obtained in the larger study for individual specialties indicated quite different patterns of satisfaction for physicians in different specialty areas. If this is also the case within the V.A., it would provide further specifications for needed changes within hospital departments. It may also be the case that certain specialists within the V.A. are satisfied with their present situation while extreme dissatisfaction is characteristic of other specialists.

It seems clear, however, that of the two tactics earlier suggested as viable methods of increasing the numbers of qualified physicians in V.A. hospitals, that of altering work setting characteristics would have a greater chance of success. The alternative of recruiting physicians with characteristics similar to those of current V.A. physicians is less attractive, particularly in light of the low satisfaction reported by physicians who have been working for the V.A. for extended periods of time. Whether the complex administrative structure of the V.A. can institute the kinds of changes which may be required is an important question which cannot be answered here. The potential positive consequences in terms of increasing quality medical care in V.A. facilities, however, appears to be well worth this challenge.

8 PSYCHOLOGICAL TYPE AND WORK-SETTING CHARACTERISTICS

Naomi Quenk, PhD

According to type theory, the observed relationships between personality type and such variables as medical specialty choice are mediated by processes whereby individuals seek out situations that maximize their opportunity to function using their preferred modes of perceiving and judging. The present study examines these hypothesized mediating processes more directly by focusing on the relationships between type and specific activities and characteristics of physician practices.

The study was based on responses from the same 477 physicians described in previous chapters who represent 14 different medical specialties including general and family practice, 11 practice organizations including various forms of private practice and a number of institutional settings, 5 community sizes and 5 states representing the five geographic regions of the country.

Data for the study consisted of responses to the Physician Work Setting Instrument (PWSI), a questionnaire designed to elicit the frequency with which physicians engage in particular medical activities as well as the extent to which a large number of factors are characteristic of their work situations. Ratings of degree of satisfaction with activities and characteristics were also obtained by having the physician indicate for each item whether he would like it to be more frequent or characteristic, less frequent or characteristic, the same, or whether it was irrelevant. The sum of items rated in each of these four ways were used as measures of overall satisfaction.

In addition to the PWSI, physicians filled out the Myers- Briggs Type Indicator. Nine physicians, or less than 2 % did not fill out the indicator. Data for this study, therefore, are based upon the responses of 468 physicians.

Data analysis in this study examined the relationship between each of the four pairs of Myers-Briggs preferences and frequency or "characteristicness" of the 62 questionnaire items, the seven clusters, and other variables judged relevant to type preferences. There is some redundancy in the data in that items included as part of clusters were also tested individually in order to present greater detail for type relationships.

The t-test for the significance of differences between means was performed on these variables, comparing extraverts to introverts, sensing types to intuitives, etc. Results are therefore for single type preferences rather than the usual combination of four preferences and are therefore not presented in type table format.

Results

Before proceeding to the results of the study, it would be helpful to be aware of the overall distribution of personality types in the sample studied. (Table 60) As can be seen, this sample does not look like samples of medical students with which we are familiar. In comparison to medical students, these physicians in practice are highly over-represented with sensing and judging types and to a lesser extent with introverts and thinking types. ISTJs represent 21% of this sample as compared to 8% of a combined medical student sample. Although a study of non-responders to the project revealed no significant differences in such variables as age, board certification, membership in specialty societies, community size and state of practice; there were some differences in response rate by medical specialty area. Pathologists were the best responders with neurosurgeons the poorest. Unfortunately, comparative type data were unavailable and it seems likely that type preferences may be related to willingness to respond to this kind of study. In addition, however, the nature of the specialties required for the larger project included a large number where sensing and judging types could be expected, such as general and family practice and five surgical specialties. In spite of the nature of this sample, however, type tables for individual specialties are generally consonant with over and under- representations previously found by Myers and Davis [80].

Table 61 shows each of the variables for which type differences occurred on one or more of the four preferences. The level of significance of the difference is indicated by asterisks. For clusters, activities and characteristics, the type preferences listed are always for the higher mean score, such that persons of that type preference indicated that the item was very frequent or very characteristic. Activities were rated on a five point scale ranging from "never" to "performed daily" while a six point scale of characteristicness was used ranging from very uncharacteristic to very characteristic.

As can be seen, introverts, sensing types and judging types are significantly older than their opposites, and intuitives tend to be more recent graduates of medical schools. These results for sensing-intuition may reflect changing medical school admissions procedures, particularly the greater influence of MCAT scores as an admissions criterion.

Sensing, thinking and judging types have remained longer in their present setting, which may be partly a function of the increased age of sensing and judging types. However, such a finding is also in line with type predictions for persons with these preferences.

That sensing types practice in smaller communities confirms previous findings by Myers and MacCaulley [81] and Quenk and Albert [82]. The higher income of sensing and judging types may be related to their age and longer time in their present setting. Again, however, type values are consonant with a greater focus on earnings for these types than for intuitives and perceptives. Sensing types see significantly more patients than intuitives, which is probably related to their preference for primary care specialties and practice in small communities, both of which are typically associated with higher patient loads.

The intuitive's preference for complexity and variety appears to be reflected in their greater likelihood of dividing their time among two or more regular work settings.

Because these data were analyzed for pairs of individual preferences, the remainder of the results will be presented by examining items which characterize each preference, rather than all of the preferences which are associated with each item. The table, however, permits this letter kind of examination of results.

Extraverts versus Introverts

Extraverts are significantly higher than introverts on cluster 1 - Personal Patient Involvement. They are also characterized by greater responsibility for defining one's role, duties and activities (item 1), personal control of amount of time devoted to patient care (item 2), dealing with patients' emotional difficulties (item 7), personally handling financial aspects of medical practice (item 20), opportunity

Table 60. Distribution of Types in Taxonomy Sample (N=468)

Sensing		Intuitive				
With Thinking	With Feeling	With Feeling	With Thinking	Type	N	%
ISTJ N = 98 % = 20.9	ISFJ N = 44 % = 9.4	INFJ N = 38 % = 8.1	INTJ N = 37 % = 7.9	E	192	41.1
				I	276	58.9
				S	247	52.8
				N	221	47.2
ISTP N = 12 % = 2.6	ISFP N = 8 % = 1.7	INFP N = 25 % = 5.3	INTP N = 14 % = 3.0	T	255	54.5
				F	213	45.5
				J	333	71.2
				P	135	28.8
ESTP N = 8 % = 1.7	ESFP N = 12 % = 2.6	ENFP N = 38 % = 8.1	ENTP N = 18 % = 3.8	IJ	217	46.4
				IP	59	12.6
				EP	76	16.2
				EJ	116	24.8
ESTJ N = 39 % = 8.3	ESFJ N = 26 % = 5.6	ENFJ N = 22 % = 4.7	ENTJ N = 29 % = 6.2	ST	157	33.5
				SF	90	19.2
				NF	123	26.3

| | | | | NT | 98 | 20.9 |

Table 61. Work Setting Characteristics in Relation to Type

Variables	E-I	S-N	T-F	J-P
Physician's age (older physicians)	I*	S***		J***
Length of time in present setting (longer time)		S***	T*	J***
Year of graduation from medical school (more recently)		N**		
Community size (smaller)		S***		
Income from medicine (higher income		S*		J**
Average number patients seen per week (greater number)		S**		
Number of regular work settings (greater number)		N**		
Cluster 1 - Personal Patient Involvement	E***		F***	
Cluster 2 - Physician teacher		N**	T**	
Cluster 4 - Medical Innovation		N**	T***	
Cluster 6 - Interaction with medical community			T*	
Cluster 7 - Professional ambition			T***	
1. Responsibility for defining one's role, duties and activities	E***		T***	
2. Personal control of amount of time devoted o patient care	E***			
3. Supervision of subordinates			F***	
4. Trying out new ideas		N**	T**	
5. Expanding one's own knowledge in an area of medicine		N**	T***	
6. Serious financial constraints limiting provision of patient care			F***	
7. Dealing with patients' emotional difficulties	E***	N**	F***	P**
8. Access to new developments in a field of interest or specialization			T*	
9. Emphasis on diagnosing and developing treatment plans			T*	
10. Maintaining a fairly consistent and predictable patient scheduling system.		S*		J*

Physician Career Choice and Satisfaction

Item	C1	C2	C3	C4	C5
11. Personal control of amount of earnings					J**
12. Access to hospital facilities					J*
13. Opportunity for affiliation with a medical school		N***	T***		
14. Focus on a special interest area within a specialty			T*		
15. Opportunity for professional advancement			T***		
16. Teaching medical students, interns or residents			T*		
17. Intellectual stimulation through interaction with colleagues					J**
18. Performing habitual or non-varying medical activities		S**			J**
19. Delegation of certain medical tasks to subordinates			T***		J*
20. Personally handling financial aspects of medical practice	E***	S*			J**
21. Opportunity to follow and evaluate patient progress	E**	N**			
22. Advising or counseling patients and/or their families	E**	N*		F***	
23. Opportunity for appreciation and prestige from the lay public	E***				
24. Accessibility of consultation services	E**	N*			
25. Isolation from other physicians	I*				P***
26. Direct patient contact				F*	
27. Opportunity for prestige and recognition from colleagues	E***		T*		
28. Time "wasted" due to travel between professional locations		N***			
29. Working with or under a community board or citizens' group	E**				P*
30. Taking less vacation and/or free time than one is entitled to take	I**				
31. Maintaining my preferred "pace of life"		S***			J*
32. Determining amount of free time and/or vacation time		S**			J***
33. Sufficient time for family and/or outside activities	E**	S*			
34. Opportunities for spouse to be employed or pursue preferred activities		N***	F**		
35. Active participation in non-medical community affairs	E***		F**		

Item	E	I	S	N	T	F	J	P
36. Case consultation with other professional personnel					T*		J***	
37. Supervision and/or teaching medical students or medical personnel (e. g., paramedics)				N**				
38. Providing some form of patient care outside of the major practice setting (e. g., community clinics, hospitals, etc.)	E**					F***		
39. Performing diagnostic procedures, including lab tests, upper G.I. series, biopsies, cytologies, autopsies, etc.					T**		J**	
40. Presenting cases to some audience				N**	T**			
41. Reviewing patient charts, including analysis of test results					T***			
42. Organizational administration (e. g., committee work, policy development)					T*			
43. Assisting other physicians in performing procedures							J**	
44. Referring patients to other practitioners or institutions	E***							
Sum of items rated irrelevant to satisfaction								P**
Sum of items M.D. wants "less characteristic"								P**
Sum of items M.D. wants "more characteristic"								P**

Significance levels *<.05 **<.01 ***<.005
N's on which comparisons are based:: E = 136 I = 269 S = 244 N = 218 T = 253 F = 210 J = 323 P = 134

to follow and evaluate patient progress (item 21), advising and/or counseling patients and their families (22), opportunity for appreciation and prestige from the lay public (23), accessibility of consultation services (24), opportunity for prestige and recognition from colleagues (27), working with or under a community board or citizens' group (29), sufficient time for family and/or outside activities (33), active participation in non-medical community affairs (35), providing some form of patient care outside of the major practice setting (36), and referring patients to other practitioners or institutions.

Introverts, in addition to having significantly lower scores on all these variables, are significantly higher on isolation from other physicians (25) and taking less vacation or free time than one is entitled to take (30).

These items which differentiate extraverts from introverts, are consonant with predictions concerning the kinds of situations which these types would seek out and the kinds of factors which would be important to them. Extraverts appear to focus on people-dealing areas both in terms of ·patient care as well as colleague relationships and family/community interaction. These factors are less characteristic of introverts who tend to be more isolated and inner-oriented in their practice styles.

Sensing Types versus Intuitives

Sensing types are significantly higher than intuitives on maintaining a fairly consistent and predictable patient scheduling system (10), performing habitual or non-varying medical activities (13), personally handling financial aspects of medical practice (20), maintaining preferred pace of life (31), determining amount of free time or vacation time (32), and sufficient time for family and outside activities (33). Intuitives, who are low scorers on these items, are significantly higher on cluster 2 - Physician Teacher, cluster 4 - Medical Innovation, trying out new ideas (item 4), expanding one's own knowledge in an area of medicine (5), serious financial constraints limiting provision of patient care (6), dealing with patients' emotional difficulties (7), opportunity for affiliation with a medical school (13), opportunity to follow and evaluate patient progress (21), advising or counseling patients or their families (22), accessibility of consultation services (24), time wasted due to travel between professional locations (26), opportunities for spouse to be employed or pursue preferred activities (34), supervision or teaching medical students and medical personnel (37), and presenting cases to some audience.

The kinds of items characterizing sensing types reflects their greater preference for routine and detail and related ability to exert control over their practice situations. Intuitives, on the other hand, do not focus on these kinds of factors but rather on those reflecting their preference for intellectual activities as in teaching and acquiring and using new knowledge. Also consonant with intuitive preferences is their focus on patient care activities oriented to emotional problems and patient follow-up.

Thinking versus Feeling Types

Of the 14 items which are highly characteristic of intuitives, seven are also highly characteristic of thinking types. As will be seen, all of these seven items reflect a greater concern with teaching and related activities. The sample of physicians who in the taxonomy of physician work settings were classified in the Medical Teacher niche, was over-represented with intuitive - thinking types.

Thus thinking types are significantly higher than feeling typos on cluster 2 - Physician Teacher and cluster 4 - Medical Innovation, as well as cluster 6 - Interaction with the Medical Community and cluster 7 -Professional Prestige. High scores on these clusters were characteristic of the Medical Teacher niche in the taxonomy. Thinking types are also higher on responsibility for defining one's role, duties and activities (1), trying out one's ideas (4), expanding one's own knowledge in an area of medicine (5), access to new developments in a field of interest or specialization (8), emphasis on diagnosing and developing treatment plans (9), opportunity for affiliation with a medical school (13), focus on a special interest area within a specialty (14), opportunity for professional advancement (15), teaching medical students, interns or residents (16), delegation of certain medical tasks to subordinates (19), opportunity for prestige and recognition from colleagues (27), case consultation with other professional personnel (36), supervision or teaching medical students or medical personnel (37), performing diagnostic procedures (39), presenting cases to some audience (40), reviewing patient charts (41) and organizational administration (42).

In addition to being low on all these variables, feeling types are characterized by higher Personal Patient Involvement (cluster 1), supervision of subordinates (3), serious financial constraints limiting provision of patient care (6), dealing with patients' emotional difficulties (7), advising or counseling patients and their families (22), direct patient contact (26), opportunities for spouse to be employed or pursue preferred activities (34), active participation in non-medical community affairs (35), and providing some form of patient care outside of the major practice setting (38).

Thinking-feeling appears to discriminate physicians not only on preferences related to intellectual pursuits, but on practice style emphases. Thinking types are more inclined to focus on logical approaches as seen in diagnosis and chart review, while feeling types are more concerned with personal aspects of patient care, and concern with patients' emotional and financial difficulties.

Judging versus Perceptive Types

Judging types appear to be better at item 10, maintaining a fairly consistent and predictable patient scheduling system, as well as at personal control of amount of earnings (11). They are higher on access to hospital facilities (12), intellectual stimulation through interaction with colleagues (17), performing habitual and non-varying medical activities (18), delegation of certain medical tasks to subordinates (19), personally handling financial aspects of medical practice (20), maintaining preferred pace of life (31), determining amount of free time or vacation time (32), case consultation with other professional personnel (36), performing diagnostic procedures (39), and assisting other physicians in performing procedures (43).

Perceptives are of course low on all these items and in addition are significantly higher on dealing with patients' emotional difficulties (7), isolation from other physicians (25), and working with or under a community board or citizens group (29). Judgment vs perception is the only preference where satisfaction measures are significantly different. Perceptives rate more items as irrelevant to satisfaction, and would like many items to be more characteristic of their situation and many items to be less characteristic of their situation.

Judging types share with sensing types some of the characteristics which reflect greater personal control over their professional lives. They also appear more inclined to be involved with other persons in conducting their practices, both colleagues and subordinates. Perceptives are less likely to focus on these aspects of practice. Their tendency to find more things "wrong" with their practice situations is probably a function of the greater propensity for seeing alternatives and their openness to change.

Other Analyses

In addition to the t-tests comparing opposite individual preferences, an attempt was made to determine which items best discriminated members of each Myers-Briggs type. Discriminant function analysis was used which compared members of each type to the remainder of the sample on all items previously described. Because the numbers of subjects in each of the types was relatively small, the results in many instances may be somewhat unreliable. In general, they do not add markedly to the information already reported for individual type preferences. By way of illustration, however, the results for the largest sample, ISTJs and the opposite type, ENFPs a re presented.

The discriminant function technique identifies those variables which maximally discriminate between two or more groups by forming linear combinations of discriminating variables. The goal in this case was to determine how each type differed uniquely from all other types. Because of the large number of variables included in this analysis, only the first five variables representing the greatest differences will be reported.

The items which most distinctly discriminate ISTJs from all other types are: low "availability of consultation services"; low "dealing with patients' emotional difficulties"; low "active participation in non-medical community affairs"; high "professional prestige" and high "opportunity to follow and evaluate patient progress."

For ENFPs, items which best discriminate are; low "focus on a special interest area within a specialty'";' high "number of regular settings"; high "working with or under a community board or citizens' group"; high "dealing with new or unusual patient problems"; and low "intellectual stimulation through interaction with colleagues."

Discussion

The activities and characteristics which have been found to be associated with differing Myers-Briggs preferences, corroborate general notions concerning the correlates of personality type. They provide a detailed rationale for observed specialty and work setting relationships which discriminate the types and indicate that composite of work attributes function together to attract physicians to different kinds of practice opportunities. Though the assumption is that physicians seek out situations which permit them to use their favorite functions, it is not known to what extent individuals in a particular work situation succeed in molding that situation to better meet their type preferences. We may hypothesize, however, that some situations are more amenable to such molding and alteration, and also that some types are more adept and willing to mold their work situations. In any event, these results indicate that physicians report variation in the characteristics of their work situations which are consonant with type preference.

One interesting lack of association is worth noting here. This is that with the exception of perceptives, who found more things wanting in their work situations, the overall measures of satisfaction were found to be unrelated to type. In particular, no type preference was found to be related to overall satisfaction as measured by the total number of items the physician indicated he would like to remain the same in his practice situation, This result supports basic notions about personality type in that there is no hypothesized relationship between type and capacity for satisfaction, assuming that individuals have more or less successfully chosen their most appropriate work niche. A difference in satisfaction would be expected only in a situation where a person was miss-matched by type with his work setting. Indeed, in the taxonomy of physician work settings previously mentioned, such a result was suggested for a niche occupied largely by primary care physicians who as a group reported the highest level of dissatisfaction compared to other niches. In terms of Myers-Briggs type, this niche was over-represented with intuitive-feeling-perceptive types, who are typically not attracted to these specialties.

This kind of exercise which sheds light on the details of type preferences and occupational variables, seems worth pursuing in detail groups of physicians as well as other occupational groups. It can not only enhance our understanding of personality type and behavior, but provide clues to work characteristics which might be altered or eliminated in order to attract a different or broader spectrum of types to health and other fields experiencing difficulties in recruitment and retention in particular settings. In addition, in light of the fact that different work characteristics appeal to different types, efforts might be directed toward providing work descriptions for potential recruits which take this into account, rather than focusing on only one set of work characteristics on the assumption that they will be appealing to all members of an occupational group. For example, "maintaining a predictable scheduling system" along with "performing non-varying activities" may be quite appealing to sensing- judging types as descriptions of a work situation, but not to intuitive-perceptives. "Trying out new ideas" and "affiliation with a medical school" should appeal to intuitive-thinking types, but not necessarily to sensing-feeling types. Thus the relationships reported here between type and work setting characteristics should, in addition to their theoretical utility, be useful to individuals concerned with occupational recruitment and career counseling.

9 ENHANCING CAREER CHOICE USING SUMMER EXTERNSHIPS

Gerald D. Otis

In the late 1960s many members of the Student American Medical Association believed that low rates of recruitment to primary care were due to the fact that, in traditional medical schools, the student experienced a very specialized approach to the patient and was deprived of exposure to a community based primary care practice and its attendant rewards. He or she was instructed by technically proficient academicians whose experience was confined mainly to teaching institutions. In order to correct this experiential deficit they proposed the Medical Education and Community Orientation Program (MECO) in 1969. The goal of the program was to retain the strength of medical student inclinations toward primary care by providing educational experiences in the practice of primary care medicine in non-academic community hospital settings; and exposing pre-clinical medical students to health programs derived from community efforts such as free clinics, nursing homes, halfway houses, service club programs, and the like. Starting in Illinois with 70 students in 26 hospitals, MECO spread to 21 states with approximately 2500 students and 400 hospitals or clinical participants over five years. It was formally integrated into the curriculum at the University of Nebraska School of Medicine.

MECO programs ranged in duration from eight to ten weeks and were adapted to the conditions of the specific setting. They could be single preceptorships with a rural general practitioner or rotations through various specialties practiced within a community hospital. The student's educational experiences might be those formally planned by his adviser (e. g., attendance at staff meetings); those that might be expected to occur but are not formally planned (e. g., learning about physician attitudes); or those that were unplanned and unanticipated (e. g., conflicts with staff members).

MECO program content was quite variable with some experiences common to all or most students, while others were shared by only a subset of those who went through the program. However, each program implemented the objectives of medical education in community practice and community orientation to local health programs. These common themes for the experience were maintained by a national supervisory body for the program composed entirely of students representing different regions of the United State, functioning with the administrative support of SAMA. They were responsive to the individual state programs through appointed student state project directors who, with the help of state hospital, medical, and family practice associations (as well as individual hospitals, physicians, and communities) developed, maintained and financed programs on a local basis.

Over the years, the approach to program evaluation changed in many respects, with questionnaires being refined and a variety of analyses being performed. Because of the heterogeneity of experience and of participants, the potential multiplicity of effects, and the desire for analysis to provide feedback for program modification (via student selection or the alteration of program characteristics), data collection included indicators of several relatively "fixed" student attributes; measures of student career dispositions and medical values before and after participating in MECO; and assessments of program characteristics and activities.

Methods

During the 1974 cycle, the five assessment devices administered to the respondents were: a biographical inventory; the Myers-Briggs Type Indicator (MBTI); the Physician Ideology Questionnaire (PIQ); the Career Rating and Preference Inventory (CRPI); and a Program Characteristics Form (PCF). The PIQ and CRPI were both developed as part of the UNM Longitudinal Study. The biographical form, MBTI, PIQ, and CRPI were administered prior to participation in the MECO projects while the PCF was administered after participation. Both PIQ and CRPI were re-administered after the MECO experience.

The PCF was specifically designed for the MECO project and was a refinement of the earlier program activities form. It included two kinds of items. The first type requested simple descriptive or descriptive-judgmental information about the respondent's MECO institution and experience. Included in this category of items were those dealing with the type and size of the institution, the size of the community in which it was located, the number of physician participants, duration of the project, frequency and duration of meetings with the program director, and percentage of time spent in various activity areas. Also included in this category were ratings (on seven-point scales) of various aspects of the participant's orientation to the institution, meetings with supervisors, and opportunities for several different kinds of experience.

The 88 variables in this first category were factor analyzed, the analysis resulting in thirteen dimensions which characterized the variation in MECO program characteristics. Short descriptions of each dimension are:

1. *Adequacy of Orientation* - The degree to which subject's presence in the institution was legitimized; persons to go to for assistance were specified; relevance of the program to subject's future role as physician was shown; subject was introduced to staff and others; roles, duties, and schedules were specified; subject was given overview of institutional operation.

2. *Adequacy of Meetings with Adviser* - The degree to which subject rated meetings with his adviser as interesting, deep, productive, clear, broad, hard (vs. easy), practical (vs. theoretical),

orderly, and frequent.

3. *Formal vs. Informal Meeting Style* - The degree to which subject rated meetings with his adviser as flexible, relaxed, and informal.

4. *Opportunity for Observational Experience* - The amount of opportunity to observe and discuss: physician roles; the organization of medical practice; physician attitudes; health care issues; family medicine; the relation of the hospital to the community; and health care patterns.

5. *Institutional Size* - The degree to which the subject's MECO institution was characterized by: a large number of beds; a large surrounding community; and a large number of participating physicians.

6. *Hospital Operation Emphasis* - The amount of time subject spent in admissions, administrative procedures, medical records, social services, and staff committees.

7. *Sub-Specialty Emphasis* - The amount of time subject spent in medical and surgical sub-specialty areas.

8. *Mental Health Emphasis* - The amount of time subject spent in mental health clinics and in alcohol and narcotics rehabilitation programs.

9. *Laboratory Procedures* - The amount of time subject spent in biochemistry, hematology and microbiology labs, and/or in the blood bank.

10. *Emphasis on Community Programs* - The amount of time subject spent in immunization, health education, pre-school and prenatal programs, and at sanitary facilities.

11. *Child Emphasis* - The amount of time spent in postpartum, ante-partum, nursery, labor room, pediatrics, and gynecology.

12. *Operations Emphasis* - The amount of time subject spent in the operating room, recovery room, and anesthesia.

13. *Community Health Facilities* - The amount of time subject spent in public health clinics or other community health facilities.

The second category of items in the PCF were ratings made by the respondents of the "success" of their MECO project. The 17 ratings in this set were also factor analyzed and resulted in four dimensions of success:

1. *Personal Success* - The degree to which the subject perceived his MECO experience to be successful in clarifying his preferences for medical work settings, type and size of community in which to practice, medical specialty, and increasing his knowledge about people.

2. *Community Orientation Success* - The degree to which the subject was inclined to return to the same or a similar community as a result of his MECO experience and the likelihood he would

recommend MECO to others.

3. *System Knowledge Success* - The degree to which the subject perceived his MECO program as increasing his knowledge about: patterns of health care delivery; the operation of health care institutions; social, cultural, economic, and political determinants of health and illness; and about communities in general.

4. *Technical-Clinical Knowledge Success* - The degree to which the respondent perceived his MECO project to increase his knowledge about technical aspects of medicine, clinical aspects of medicine, medical practice in general, and about the different specialties in medicine.

The dependent variables that were indexed via the assessment devices thus included 4 dimensions of program success as perceived by participants; changes in 4 dimensions of physician ideology; and changes in dispositions toward 10 specialty areas, 16 practice organizations, 8 classes of professional activity, 6 geographic locations and 5 community sizes. The independent variables included 20 background characteristics; 4 personality indexes; pre-program scores on the 4 physician ideology dimensions and 44 career dispositions; and 13 program characteristics dimensions plus program duration and specialty of program adviser. Data was provided for the analysis by 420 pre-clinical medical students who participated in MECO projects in 21 states during the summer of 1973. Sixteen percent of the respondents were female, 19 percent were married, and the mean age was 23 years.

Multiple-regression analysis was the statistical technique selected to evaluate the relative direct contributions to the determination of perceived success from variables in the student-characteristics domain and the program-characteristics domain. This procedure is most easily viewed in terms of prediction: multiple regression produces a linear combination of independent variables which are weighted so as to maximize the correlation with a dependent variable while taking into account the inter-correlations among the independent variables. When all the variables are normalized, the magnitude of the weights assigned to the independent variables in the prediction equation (the Beta weights) reflect the strength and direction of the direct relationship between independent and dependent variables. Four regression equations were calculated, one for each of the success dimensions, using the same set of independent variables.

Results

The largest single contribution to the prediction of *Personal Success* (i.e., success in clarifying career preferences) came from subjects' initial dispositions towards family medicine: the greater the inclination towards family medicine, the greater the degree of personal success. About the same level of effect came from size of high school (the smaller the school, the more the success), Community Orientation on the PIQ, and initial preference levels for psychiatry, solo practice and work in educational institutions. Among the program characteristics variables, informal meeting styles and an emphasis on mental health programs exerted the greatest positive effects while the amount of time spent in laboratory tended to reduce personal success. Maximum multiple correlation was 0.700.

The largest single contribution to the prediction of *Community Orientation Success* (subject's report of inclination to return to the same or a similar community to practice) was attraction to work in an educational institution: the more attracted to work in such settings, the less likely the subject would report wanting to return to his MECO community or one like it. Substantial contributions to prediction of this type of success also came from the number of female siblings in respondent's family (the fewer sisters, the more success); presence or absence of prior work experience in medical settings or in technical-research areas (the greater success occurred *without* such experience); relative amount of dis-preference for technique-and-instrument oriented specialties (ophthalmology, otolaryngology, radiology, etc,). solo and mixed specialty group practice; and relative amount of preference for surgery and work in industry or research. Program characteristics which contributed to success were: degree of orientation adequacy, amount of exposure to community programs (a lack of exposure going with greater success), and amount of exposure to activities in the operating and recovery rooms. Maximum multiple correlation was 0.810.

System Knowledge Success had, as its best single predictor, the subject's initial preference for working in government institutions or agencies. Almost as great contributions came from initial preference for family medicine and the adequacy of meetings with MECO advisers. System Knowledge Success scores tended to be higher for subjects who graduated from smaller high schools, who lacked prior technical or research experience, who's mothers were of higher occupational status, and who were of a "Thinking" orientation on the MBTI. High scorers were inclined to dislike the basic sciences, physical medicine and rehabilitation, and work in military type settings while being attracted to work in health departments and institutions. Program characteristics which contributed to success were adequacy of orientation, opportunity for observational experience, time spent in observing the operation of the hospital and program duration. Maximum multiple correlation was 0.740.

Technical-Clinical Knowledge Success was best predicted by the size of the MECO institution: the larger the institution, the more the success. Success scores tended to be higher if the respondent was single, had fewer male siblings, came from a small high school and had experience in dealing with the public (e. g., as a salesman). High scores on the Physician Authority scale (PIQ), more adequate meetings with the MECO adviser, greater opportunity for observational experience, more exposure to internal medicine and surgery sub-specialties, more time in lab and surgical operations and less time in mental health areas, all contributed to higher success scores. Maximum multiple correlation was 0.730.

As judged by the number of coefficients over +/- . 09, the first three types of success appear to be about equally affected by variables in the student-characteristics domain. Only Technical-Clinical Knowledge Success stands out as being relatively less affected by such variables. Program characteristics variables yielded about the same number of coefficients over +/- .09 for each type of success. The variables that entered into the regression equations for three or more types of success with coefficients greater than +/- 09 were: size of high school; technical-research experience; number of male siblings; Physician Authority; initial preferences for family medicine, surgery, and work in government institutions or agencies; and the program characteristics of Orientation Adequacy, Opportunity for Observational Experience, Mental Health Emphasis, Laboratory Emphasis and Operations Emphasis. Variables that appeared to be irrelevant to any of the four types of success (having Beta coefficients less than +/-.09) were: age, sex, importance of religion, experience in "helping" activities or teaching, Introversion (MBTI). Empathy and Rapport with Patients (PIQ), Psychosocial Orientation (PIQ), initial preferences for obstetrics-gynecology, pediatrics, work in a medical team, large group practice, or for the Public Health Service.

Discussion

The results indicate that a substantial amount of variance in participants' success ratings of their MECO experiences can be accounted for by the person characteristics and program characteristics here assessed. If one were to accept as the objective of the MECO project the maximizing of participants' experience of one or more of the four types of success, the findings could be fed back into the administrative decision-making process at two points: the selection of participants and the design of MECO programs. For example, in order to increase the amount of Community Orientation Success, it would be desirable to give preference to students who have not had previous experience in medical care settings (other things being equal). Or, in order to increase the amount of Technical-Clinical Knowledge Success, it would be desirable to assign students to only the larger institutions available.

Manipulation of some variables would tend to increase (or decrease) the experienced success in all four areas. For example, selection of students from small high school graduating classes would, according to this analysis, increase Personal, Community Orientation, System Knowledge and Technical-Clinical Success; and focusing of program advisers' attention on the importance of orientation experiences and the opportunity for observational experience might increase success in several domains. However, with some variables, an increase in experienced success of one type would be accompanied by a decrease in experienced success of another type. This is the case with technical-research experience, the presence of which increases Personal Success but decreases Community Orientation and System Knowledge Success. Likewise, increasing the amount of time students spend in mental health areas could be expected to increase Personal Success but decrease Community Orientation and Technical-Clinical Knowledge Success. Consideration of these probable conflicting effects would thus require the decision makers to either (1) abandon the identified variable as one to be manipulated, or (2) prioritize their success objectives, (i. e., decide which type of success is more important.)

It should be noted that the method of analysis used in this study imposes certain restrictions on the interpretation of the results. First of all, it ignores indirect effects, (i. e., the effects of one variable on another operating through an intervening variable); for example, in the present study the effects of personality variables on experienced success were found, for the most part, to be minor. Yet, it is known from other studies that personality variables have effects on specialty and practice organization preferences. They could thus, indirectly affect success through their effects on career preferences. Path analysis, which requires specification of hypothesized relationships between variables, could obtain estimates of the magnitude of such indirect effects.

Secondly, the method forces a "linear compensatory", model on the data. The phrase "other things being equal" tacked on to the interpretation of the effects of a variable means that its effects can be overshadowed by the values which an individual obtains on other variables. Thus, graduation from a large high school can be compensated for by having a stronger than average inclination towards family practice.

Finally, non-linear relations between independent and dependent variables and interaction effects are not represented in the analysis. This is not really a restriction of the method, however, since they could be included by generating "hybrid" variables. This was not done because of the large numbers of possible combinations of variables and the absence of very good rationale for reducing their number.

In spite of these drawbacks, the results may be considered a good first approximation to evaluation of the relative contributions of a large number of variables to participants' perceived success in a complex educational experience. It remains for future research and analysis to identify other relevant variables, refine their indexes, and detail the causal relationships involved.

Methods 2

In this assessment the MBTI was dropped from the previous list of questionnaires while retaining the other questionnaires. 526 cases were added and data analysis focused on four areas: student characteristics, program characteristics, program outcomes, and selected breakdowns. The first two areas are largely descriptive, dealing with the nature of MECO participants and MECO projects. The next section, program outcomes, considers how participants judged the success of their projects and assesses differences in pre-MECO and post-MECO attitudes and career dispositions. The last section, selected breakdowns, is the most interesting from a researcher's point of view. It looks at measures of "program success" and changes in career dispositions as a function of certain student characteristics and program characteristics.

Student Background Characteristics

Perusal of the percentage distributions for background characteristics gave few indications that MECO participants were much different from other medical students. The "typical" MECO· respondent was male, 23 years old, single, Caucasian and Protestant. His father was an executive, professional or administrator and his mother was a housewife. He was the oldest child in a relatively large family (three boys, one girl), majored in one of the biological sciences as a college student and minored in a physical science. Prior to entering medical school he had occupational or organizational experience in more than one of the following: medical settings, "helping" activities, research-technology, teaching, and dealing with the public. The only obvious biases in comparison with the population of medical students appears to be in the geographic origin of MECO respondents: they were mainly from the Midwest and from non-metropolitan areas.

Initial Career Dispositions

The mean values obtained for ratings of initial career dispositions suggest that the "typical" MECO participant planed to become a family practitioner (or perhaps specialize in internal medicine) and practice in a group arrangement, preferably with a mixture of specialists. His geographic preference (for the Midwest) corresponded to his region of origin although the Rocky Mountain area had much appeal. In terms of community size, his preference was for small town living. These dispositions are in marked contrast to the specialty and geographic distribution of physicians in practice. However, in comparison with students at the same stage of medical education at one medical school (UNM) which used the same rating scales, the differences were not so dramatic. Nevertheless, there seemed to be some differences even when these comparisons were made. MECO respondents were initially more inclined than UNM medical students (1st and 2nd yr.) toward family medicine, group (and especially team) practice, and work in an industrial setting or for an independent medical foundation. Initial career dispositions were lower for MECO respondents for pediatrics, psychiatry, solo practice, work in government institutions, private hospitals and educational institutions and for practice in a metropolitan area.

From what comparative evidence exists, then, MECO participants in 1975 appeared to be "biased" in that they tended to come from smaller communities and have career dispositions toward family practice in small communities. As will be seen below, these characteristics are probably interrelated. (It should be remembered, of course, that generalizations from modal frequencies and averages taken one at a time disregard combinations of attributes and all of those non-modal cases which, combined, may exceed the mode. Thus, the picture drawn above may be quite distorted for many MECO respondents.)

Program Characteristics: Orientation, Supervision, Observational Experience, Dimensions

Most MECO projects took place in general hospitals with an average bed size of 200 An average of 13 physicians actively participated in the MECO program and nearly half of the program advisers were family practitioners. During the average nine weeks of the program students spent the largest proportion of their time (about 25%) in areas dealing with surgical operations, i.e. the operating and recovery rooms, anesthesiology and radiology. The next greatest proportions of time were spent in sub-specialty areas (18%) and birth, infant and child care areas (14%). Of the seven areas assessed, the least time was spent in the area of mental health programs (3%).

On the average, orientations to MECO projects were rated between "satisfactory" and "extremely well done" by the 1975 respondents. The aspects of orientation perceived to be most adequately carried out were: introducing the student to other staff with whom he would work; specifying who the student was to go to for information and assistance; and showing the relevance of the program to the student's future role as a physician. Those aspects least well performed were in specification of program goals and specification of student roles or duties. The form that MECO projects assumed were negotiated with the program director in most cases.

The frequency of supervision varied considerably with weekly sessions being the mode. Thirty-one percent of the respondents met with their supervisor for an hour or more while 41% met for 15 minutes or less each session. Sixty five percent characterized these meetings as "quite productive" or "extremely productive and enriching." Topics during these meetings tended to be characterized as broad, practical, clinical, and biological and of interest to students. A "psychosocial" orientation did not appear prominent since ratings tended toward the opposite pole of "socially oriented," "behavioral," and "community based." In other words, clinical medicine seemed to be the major focus.

The style of supervisory sessions was characterized by the 1975 respondents as relaxed, clear, informal, flexible and oriented to student projects. Thus, it appears students had a good deal of influence in determining the course of these sessions.

Most students felt they had a lot of opportunity to observe and discuss the roles and attitudes of practicing physician and family practice; and a fair amount of opportunity to observe and discuss the organization of medical practice, health care patterns and issues, medical staff structure and the relations of the hospital to the community. The only area that appeared to be slighted was the nature of allied health roles.

Data analyses carried out in prior years had indicated that most of these ratings of program characteristics could be reduced to 13 "program characteristic" dimensions on the basis of inter- correlations between the various items of information. Scores on each of the 13 dimensions (which are largely independent of one another) could then be computed for each individual to take the place of the much larger set of individual item ratings. Results of dimensional analysis with the new data was the same as in the previous year. Compared to the MECO programs of 1974, those of 1975 showed a significant decrease in emphasis on Hospital Operations (f), Community Health Programs (j), Community Health Facilities (m) and Child Care (k). The Adequacy of Meetings with Adviser (b), however, showed a significant increase from 1974. It is difficult to tell just what this means although it might be hypothesized that these differences reflect a movement away from more socially and community oriented concerns and toward more practical career interests.

Program Characteristics and Hospital Size

The largest hospitals (401 + beds) had their MECO students spend more time in birth areas than did other hospitals and less time in surgical operations. Time spent in sub-specialty areas appeared to be curvilinearly related to hospital size with a maximum in hospitals of 201-300 beds. With the exception of hospitals in the 301-400 bed category, time spent in lab decreased with increasing hospital size as did time spent in learning about the operation of hospital.

Adequacy of orientation was poorest for the very large hospitals as was the opportunity for observational experience. As was indicated by the percentage of time figures, the emphasis on hospital operations, laboratory procedures, community programs and surgical operations were all decreasing functions of hospital size. Sub-specialty emphasis and mental health emphasis both showed the lowest scores at the extremes of hospital size, i. e., either 100 beds and below or 401 beds and above.

With a few exceptions these relationships are quite similar to those found in previous years . What they probably reflect are different structures of operation and values in hospitals of different sizes and their consequences in terms of educational opportunities for MECO participants. These differences should be evaluated in terms of program goals and the relationships of program characteristics to program outcomes (see the section on selected breakdowns).

Program Outcomes: Student Perceptions of Program Success

Mean judgments of program success ranged between "slightly successful" to "very successful" depending upon the objective being rated. The most highly rated objectives were: increasing knowledge about the organization and operation of health care institutions; people in general; medical practice, in general; and clarifying preferences for a type or size community in which to practice. Least highly rated (although still close to "moderately successful") were: increasing knowledge about the different specialties in medicine and about the functions and skills of allied health personnel.

Nearly all students reported they would recommend MECO to others; 90% said they would be interested in returning to a similar community to practice and 78% would be interested in returning to the same community ; and 83% of the respondents would suggest the hospital be used as an elective. Dimensional analysis of success judgments yielded the same four clusters as previously: Personal Success, Community Orientation Success, System Knowledge Success and Technical-clinical Knowledge Success. Compared to 1974, scores on these "success dimensions" all increased for 1975. However, none of the increases were large enough to be considered statistically significant.

Program Outcomes: Attitude Changes

The four medical attitudes assessed pre-MECO and post-MECO were:

a) <u>Empathy and Rapport with Patients</u>: the value placed on a physician being able to put patients at ease; being warm, understanding, reassuring, dignified and tactful with patients; the importance of exploring reasons for a patient's non-compliance, of not keeping patients waiting, and of having knowledge of a patient's family situation.

b) <u>Psychosocial Orientation</u>: the value placed on team work to treat or deal with the psychological and social problems of patients. According to the high scorer, the ideal physician would apply his knowledge of psychosocial medicine, psychiatry and psychosomatic medicine in the clinical practice of medicine. He would know the skills of non-medical specialists and work with them in a team setting and he would be acquainted with the social and welfare agencies in his community so that he could deal with some of the social problems of patients. He would have skill in interpersonal relations, explore social and emotional factors when taking a history, be oriented to the long-term care of patients, and adapt treatment to their special needs or circumstances.

c) <u>Community Orientation</u>: the value attached to the physician being involved in professional activities in the community -- being a leader in health planning, reserving time for community service, participating in community heath programs.

d) <u>Physician Authority</u>: the value placed upon a physician having control over patient care and his work setting and of patients following orders.

For the total group of MECO respondents for 1975, only the Physician Authority scale showed a statistically significant change (an increase). Data from the University of New

Mexico Longitudinal Study indicate that scores on this scale generally increase over time in medical school so that the change observed here may not be an effect due to MECO. It might be hypothesized, however, that hospital experience during pre-clinical years accelerates the increase.

Program Outcomes: Changes in Career Dispositions

Statistically significant *decreases* occur for dispositions toward: physical medicine and rehabilitation, psychiatry, public health, work in industrial settings, in independent foundations and in research institutions. Statistically significant *increases* occur for team practice and work in educational and non-government institutions, especially private hospitals. All other pre-MECO to post-MECO changes were not statistically significant.

In order to have some standard by which to judge these changes (and non-changes), the trends were compared to trends in the University of New Mexico sample. For the most part, changes or lack of changes in MECO ratings corresponded to changes or lack of changes in UNM ratings. There were a few exceptions, however. Students at UNM tended to show a decrease in inclination toward family practice (vs. no change for 1975 MECO respondents); UNM students increased in psychiatry disposition (vs. a decrease for MECO); UNM students remained constant in their disposition toward public health (vs a decrease for MECO); UNM students showed a decrease in disposition toward working in the VA or a military hospital (vs. constant for MECO); UNM students did not show the increase in preference for team practice until the third year of medical school; UNM students decreased in preference for government sponsored health programs and work in the public health service (vs. no change in MECO respondents); UNM students did not show any change in disposition toward industry, independent foundations and research as did MECO respondents; and preference for work in educational institutions remained constant in UNM students (vs. an increase for MECO respondents).

For the work setting data, the differences between UNM students and MECO participants appear to be captured by the term "regression toward the mean". That is, where MECO respondents were initially above or below the mean for UNM students, they "moved" to values corresponding to the UNM mean values. For example, MECO respondents initially rated work in education institutions as less attractive than UNM students but increased in their disposition toward such work settings by the end of their MECO experiences. What this phenomenon means in a substantive sense, if anything, is unclear at this point.

For the specialty preference data, the "regression toward the mean" phenomena does not seem to hold. MECO respondents were initially more disposed toward family practice and stayed so disposed while UNM students tend to reduce their family practice preference. And for psychiatry, MECO respondents were less disposed than UNM students and decreased their preference even further by the end of their preceptorships. UNM students, on the other hand, tended to increase their preference for psychiatry.

It should be remembered that the above results are overall results, disregarding differences in program characteristics and types of students. What they indicate is that the net changes in specialty dispositions associated with students taking MECO preceptorships are slight while the net changes in certain practice organization dispositions may be significant. Changes for particular types of students and particular kinds of MECO programs may indeed be significant (and consistent) in spite of the lack of substantial overall changes. This is shown to some extent in the selected breakdowns reported in the next section of this report but deserves to be investigated further.

Selected Breakdowns by Student Characteristics and Program Characteristics

Marital status, high school community size, sex and father's occupational status were unrelated to any of the four types of perceived program success.

Individuals with prior work experience in medical settings perceived significantly less personal, system knowledge and technical-clinical knowledge success, perhaps because they had less to learn than students without such experience. Students with undergraduate majors in the biological or physical sciences perceived significantly less technical-clinical knowledge success than did students who majored in the social sciences, humanities or engineering. Protestants seemed to perceive more community orientation success than other religious groups or those with no religious affiliation. And first born children perceived greater success in all areas except community orientation success.

Breakdown of success scores according to program characteristics indicated that those students who had their programs in large metropolitan areas perceived less personal and system knowledge success than those who went to small or medium size towns while students in medium size cities experienced the most technical-clinical knowledge success.

Individuals who had radiologists as program directors perceived the greatest personal and technical-clinical knowledge success while those with pediatrician directors perceived the least.

Mean scores on the four success dimensions as a function of hospital size (in beds) show that for personal and system knowledge success, scores tended to decrease with increasing hospital size. Hospitals over 300 beds tended to have less community orientation success while technical-clinical knowledge success was the poorest at both extremes of hospital size. These relationships are similar to those found in previous years. Selection of hospitals in the 100 to 200 bed range would appear to maximize the perceived success in most areas.

With respect to career dispositions, a breakdown of preference for family practice by specialty of the program director (family physicians vs. all others) and stage (pre-MECO vs. post-MECO) revealed that those who were directed by family physicians were initially more inclined toward family practice. However, over the course of their MECO experiences the two groups diverged with those directed by family physicians increasing their preference for family practice and those directed by other types of physicians (specialists) decreasing their preference for family practice. One would suppose this effect to be due to some kind of "role modeling".

Three-way breakdowns were performed on family practice dispositions and preference for practice in small towns using size of high school community, size of MECO community and stage as the independent variables. The family practice disposition breakdown showed that: (1) disposition toward family practice was inversely related to size of home town both before and after MECO; (2) size of home town, by itself, did not affect *change* in dispositions toward family practice; (3) size of MECO community was linearly related to disposition toward family practice prior to MECO but curvilinearly related after MECO (with the medium size cities showing the least preference); (4) only placement in medium size cities had a significant effect on the amount of change in disposition toward family practice (decreasing it) and this held for all sizes of home town. Thus, the end result was that small town students placed in small towns for their MECO projects had the highest post-MECO dispositions toward family practice; and those students from metropolitan areas or medium size cities who were placed in medium size cities had the lowest post-MECO dispositions toward family practice.

The corresponding three-way breakdown using dispositions toward practicing in small towns as the dependent variable produced somewhat similar results. (l) Small town students, initially and post-MECO, had greater dispositions toward practicing in small towns ; (2) placement in medium size cities decreased preference for practicing in small towns but placement in metropolitan areas tended to increase preference for small towns; (3) placement in small towns increased the preference for practicing in small towns for students from medium size cities and from metropolitan areas but not the preference of those from small towns. The resulting post-MECO preferences for practicing in small towns were highest for small town students placed in large cities and students from medium size cities placed in small towns, the lowest post -MECO scores were for metropolitan students placed in metropolitan areas or medium size cities.

The results suggest that placement in small towns for individuals who have never lived in such communities can be a "turn on" and that placement in large metropolitan areas for individuals who have not spent a great deal of time in such communities can be a "turn off". Why placement in medium size cities tends to reduce preference for small communities in students from metropolitan areas is not so clear. Perhaps the medium size cities "recruit" metropolitan students for themselves thereby diminishing preference for practice in smaller communities.

Finally, the beta coefficients for each program characteristic dimension obtained when they were used to predict the different kinds of perceived program success were examined. The size and sign of these coefficients indicate the magnitude and direction of the relationship to the success measures. Since the same variables and the same methods were used in each regression run, the coefficients may be compared both within and across success dimensions.

A high degree of informality in student meetings with their advisers was the program characteristic most strongly associated with Personal Success while it showed very minor relationships to other types of success. Opportunity for observational experience was most predictive of both System Knowledge Success and Technical-clinical Knowledge Success. Emphasis on Hospital Operation appeared to help System Knowledge Success but decrease Technical-clinical Knowledge Success. (The results for Community Orientation Success had best be disregarded since there was very little variability in scores on that dimension).

The best predictions from program characteristics was for <u>System Knowledge Success</u> with the highest weights from Observational Experience, Orientation Adequacy and Hospital Operation. <u>Personal Success</u> was best predicted from Informality of Meetings, Observational Experience, Orientation Adequacy and Surgical Operations. <u>Technical-clinical Knowledge Success</u> was most significantly influenced by Observational Experience, Sub-specialty Experience and Surgical Operations. <u>Community Orientation Success</u> was poorly predicted, again because there was little variability in the scores (nearly everyone endorsed the relevant items).

The results of this analysis show that the *program characteristics* important for one or more types of success are: Orientation Adequacy, Hospital Operation Emphasis, Sub-specialty Emphasis, Opportunity for Observational Experience, Informal Meeting Style, Adequacy of Meetings and Surgical Operations Emphasis.

Addendum: Effects of Preceptorship Location on Medical Student Dispositions Toward Small Town Practice

The problem of physician scarcity in non-metropolitan areas of the United States has been linked to, among other things, the nature of the educational milieu in medical schools [82, 83, 84]. Training experiences which occur for the most part in urban university medical centers and emphasize specialization and research are believed to discourage students from entering general and family practice and from practicing in locations without the most up-to-date facilities.

One approach to the modification of medical student educational experiences has been the development of preceptorship programs in medically under-served areas[85, 86, 87]. These programs have emerged in most areas of the country, many sponsored by medical schools and supported under the Comprehensive Health Manpower Training Act of 1971 as amended by PL92-157; others have been sponsored by professional groups or student organizations.

Attempts to assess the effects of such programs on student dispositions toward rural or small town practice have produced equivocal results. For example, Steinwald and Steinwald [88] found 28% of physicians who participated in rural training programs chose rural practice settings (versus 16% of non-participants). But most of those physicians who chose rural locations grew up in rural areas, a factor which has been found to predispose physicians toward practice in such locations [89]. Thus, both selection of rural preceptorship experiences and selection of rural practice locations could be due to an orientation engendered by growing up in non-metropolitan areas. Furthermore, participants in one preceptorship program [90] indicated on a follow-up questionnaire that their preceptorship experiences played no part in their location decisions.

Data collected as part of an assessment of the American Medical Student Association Foundation's project MECO (Medical Education and Community Orientation) provided an opportunity to examine in greater detail the relationships among size of community of origin, size of preceptorship community, and initial and subsequent dispositions toward practice in small communities.

Analysis of Dispositions Toward Small Town Practice

Before and after participation in MECO, students in the 1973, 1974, and 1975 cohorts were asked to indicate the degree of their preference or dis-preference for practicing in communities of various sizes on seven-point approach-avoidance scales. (A rating of 1 indicated the subject was "strongly inclined to avoid" the community while a rating of 7 indicated the subject was "strongly inclined to select" the community as a practice site). Data were also available on the size of the communities in which they spent their high school years and the size of the communities in which they took their MECO preceptorships. The latter were collapsed into three population categories: 100,000 or greater (metropolitan area); 25,000 to 100,000 (medium city); and less than 25,000 (small town).

Preliminary examination of the mean preference scores obtained by the nine high school community size by MECO community size groups, when rating the pre-MECO attractiveness of practice in small towns (populations of 10,000 or less), revealed significant (p<.001) associations between initial preference levels and both size of high school community and size of MECO community. In addition, the unequal number of cases in each group indicated an association between size of high school community and size of community to which assigned for preceptorship experience. This confounding of the sources of variance would make interpretation of the results of a classical analysis of variance difficult, at best.

Path analysis [91, 92, 93] seemed to provide a more suitable approach to unraveling the interrelationships of these variables. The basic idea behind path analysis is the notion that variables can be arranged in terms of causal priorities so that, when focusing upon the interrelationships within one set of variables, it is possible to ignore variables that are dependent upon the given set. The path diagram is a visual representation of this assumed flow of cause and effect. In the path diagram shown in Figure 1, the arrows indicate the direct influence of one variable upon another and the lines from the e_i represent

residual paths from all other influences on the variable in question, including errors of measurement, causes that were not recognized, and departures from additivity and linearity.

The numerical values alongside the arrows are path coefficients and represent the magnitude of expected change in one variable for a unit change in another variable, given the point of view represented in the diagram. Path coefficients are similar to partial regression coefficients but are embedded within a system that involves residuals (and sometimes other unmeasured hypothetical variables). They have meaning only when attached to a particular diagram.

In the present case, with four variables, there are 64 possible causal structures which could be examined. Most of these arrangements can be eliminated as either being trivial (e. g., zero, one, or two causal arrows) or violating the obvious time ordering of the variables. Three, four, and five arrow models, while more parsimonious than the full-scale (six arrow) model, can be revealed through path analysis of the latter by the appearance of zero-order path coefficients. Thus, the only structure that need be subjected to path analysis is that shown in Figure 2.

According to this diagram, size of community of origin (V_1) is assumed to directly influence: initial dispositions toward practice in small towns (V_2); size of the MECO community negotiated by the student (V_3); and the effects of the experience as reflected in subsequent small town practice dispositions (V_4). Initial practice dispositions are postulated to affect the size of the MECO community which was negotiated (via a motivation to "explore the role") as well as subsequent practice dispositions. And size of MECO community is seen as directly influencing the outcome of the preceptorship experience.

Estimation of parameters from correlational data in simple recursive path models, such as this one, is based on the decomposition of covariance. That is, the observed correlation between two variables is assumed to be the sum of the contributions associated with each of the elementary paths between the two variables. These elementary paths include direct links between the variables (direct effects); links between the variables that are mediated by one or more variables (indirect effects); and "backward links" where the variables have in common one or more prior variables (spurious correlation). Thus, the correlation between V_2 and V_4 in Figure 1 is equal to p42 (direct effect) plus p32* p43 (indirect effect) plus p21*p41 + p21*p31*p43 (spurious correlation). The complete set of equations that describe the model in Figure 2 are:

r21= p21

r31= p31 + p21*p32

r41= p41 + p21*p42 + p21*p32*p43 + p31*p43 r32= p32 + p21*p31

r42= p42 + p32*p43 + p21*p41 + p21*p31*p43 r43= p43 + p42*p32 + p31*p41 + p31* p 21*p42

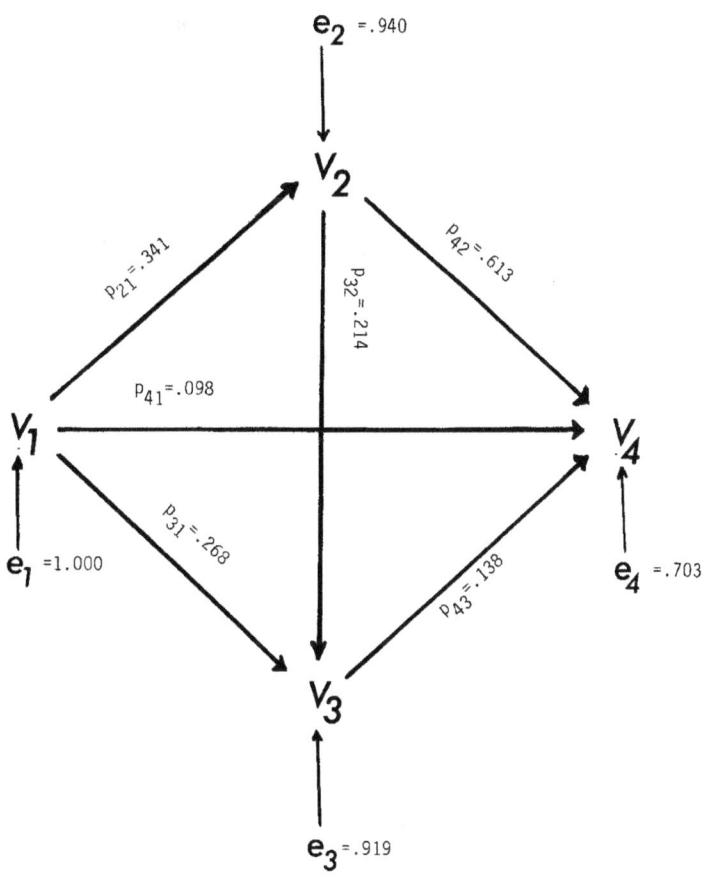

Since p21 is the correlation between V_1 and V_2, the problem reduces to five equations with four unknowns and one can solve for the values of the path coefficients using observed correlations. Figure 2. Path diagram showing the relationships among size of high school community (V_1), size of MECO community (V_3), initial dispositions toward small town practice (V_2), and subsequent dispositions toward small town practice (V_4).

This model is a special case of path analysis in which there are no unmeasured variables, residuals are uncorrelated, there is one way causation assumed, and each of the dependent variables is directly related to all variables preceding it in sequence. The path coefficients are then identical with the beta coefficients obtained through a sequence of conventional regression analyses. Thus, for the 1012 cases having complete data, V_4 was regressed on V_1, V_2, and V_3 to obtain p41, p42, and p43; and V_3 was regressed on V_2 and V_1 to obtain p32 and p31. The resulting standardized path coefficients, shown in Figure 1, were all highly significant and at least twice the size of their standard errors.

Table 62 shows the decomposition of bivariate covariation for each relationship in the model. The first thing to be noted about the results is that a little more than half of the variance in post-MECO dispositions toward small town practice was accounted for by the other three variables. Most of this was attributable to the direct effect of initial practice dispositions, i. e., those students who were initially strongly inclined toward small town practice tended to remain so inclined.

Table 62 Direct, Indirect and Total Effects for Bivariate Relationships in the Model

Relationship	Total Covariance	Casual Effect		
		Direct	Indirect	Total
V1V2	0.341	0.341	None	0.341
V1V3	0.341	0.268	0.073	0.341
V1V4	0.354	0.098	0.256	0.354
V2V3	0.305	0.214	None	0.214
V2V4	0.689	0.613	0.030	0.643
V1V4	0.358	0.138	None	0.138

Size of high school community appeared to exert the major portion of its effect indirectly by influencing initial practice dispositions and the size of the MECO community which was negotiated. Although size of MECO community had a greater direct effect on post-MECO practice dispositions than did size of high school community, the latter variable's total effect was greater.

Discussion

Results of the path analysis seem to indicate, then, that geographic location of preceptorship experiences (whether in urban or rural sites) does indeed influence dispositions toward small town practice. However, these effects may not be readily apparent in net before-after results for they are easily overshadowed by other factors. For example, if MECO were to somehow succeed in increasing the percentage of students placed in small towns by 17% (without disturbing anything else), one would expect a .085 increase in mean post-MECO ratings of small town practice. But if the proportion of preceptees who were from small communities decreased at the same time by only seven percent, this expected increase would be canceled out. A similar cancellation would occur if the mean pre-MECO ratings for small town practice dropped by only .07 points.

The example above assumes that only the values of the variables are changed and that the structure of relationships between variables remains constant. Real world manipulations, however, may affect the parameters of the model as well. Thus, in order to increase the percentage of students assigned to small towns, it might be necessary to pay less attention to student desires regarding the location of their preceptorships. The result could be a reduction in the magnitude of the "negotiation parameters" (p31 and p32). If they dropped to zero, the significance of size of community of origin in the determination of post-preceptorship dispositions toward small town practice would be reduced by 13% since two of its three indirect causal effects would be lost.

The model presented here deals only with the short-term effects of preceptorship location on medical student dispositions toward small town practice. Considering the fact that these experiences constitute only about three percent of the student's total training time and occur from three to seven years before an actual commitment to a location must be made, it would be surprising if any effects on ultimate location decisions could be detected.

In order to fairly assess the significance of these early experiences and dispositions for later choice of practice location, one should view them in terms of a much more elaborate model. Such a model might include, among other things, experiential influences which impinge upon the individual during his subsequent training; educational choices which determine the individual's exposure to different kinds of influence; and the economic, social, and professional development incentives[4] which may or may not exist at the time of "final" decision making. When viewed within this expanded context, the effect of preceptorship location on ultimate practice location decisions would probably turn out to be largely indirect, exerting its influence through a number of mediating variables.

Gerald Otis and Naomi Quenk

10 FINAL WORDS

Gerald D. Otis

The studies reported above indicate that personality and attitudinal characteristics are differentially associated with selection of medical specialty, practice organization and size of community in which to practice and that these associations hold for a considerable period of time. Furthermore, students destined for careers in Family Practice can be predicted from their entry-level dispositions toward a range of specialties with a good deal of accuracy while the fate of students not so-inclined is less certain. Similarly, students more likely to practice in institutional settings can be ascertained with reasonable accuracy from their preferences at the time they enter medical school but those slated for individual or group practices are more problematic. Most students know the size of community in which they will practice from the beginning of their medical careers. While most of those practicing in small towns come from larger communities, the *probability* that a student from a small town will end up practicing in a small town is greater than for a student whose origins are in a larger community. Physicians who teach Family Medicine, while they may share certain personality characteristics with their residents, are different from them in certain respects.

In general, satisfied physicians enjoy having challenging work, collaborating and/or having available the expertise of other health professionals, not working alone, having a satisfactory personal life for spouse and family, sharing acquired knowledge through supervision and teaching, controlling the amount they can earn and earning a higher income. While there are a large number of variables that are associated with physician satisfaction in various specialties and niches, predictability is much greater when physicians are considered with regard to their specialties and practice organizations. Variance accounted for ranged from 16% for physicians as a whole to 65% for Family Practitioners considered by themselves. Things that make for greater satisfaction in one specialty or work-setting, may make for greater dissatisfaction in another. Nearly all the variance in 25 physicians practicing in non-governmental hospitals was explained by their scores on just 9 variables. Some settings, such as V.A. Hospitals pose special problems for physician satisfaction and the factors that are important for full-time staff may be different than for part-time staff. While physicians reported variation in the characteristics of their work situations that are consonant with known Psychological Type (MBTI) preferences, overall measures of satisfaction were found to be unrelated to type. The one exception to this rule was that Perceptive Types found more things wanting in their work situations than did Judging Types.

Summer externship programs in which medical students are placed in community hospitals with a physician preceptor, can have significant effects on medical attitudes and career dispositions. Four dimensions of success were identified in these programs :*Personal Success* (clarifying his/her preferences for medical work settings, type and size of community in which to practice, medical specialty, and increasing his knowledge about people); *Community Orientation Success (*inclination to return to the same or a similar community increased); *System Knowledge Success (*increased knowledge about: patterns of health care delivery; the operation of health care institutions; social, cultural, economic, and political determinants of health and illness); and *Technical-Clinical Knowledge Success* (increased knowledge about technical and clinical aspects of medicine, medical practice in general, and about the different specialties in medicine). Success in these different domains was dependent on both program characteristics and student characteristics. Factors favoring success in one domain might favor failure in another domain. Post program dispositions toward small town practice were seen to be a function of size of community of origin, size of program community and initial dispositions toward small town practice. Size of high school community appeared to exert the major portion of its effect indirectly by influencing initial practice dispositions and the size of the program community that was negotiated. Although size of program community had a greater direct effect on post-program practice dispositions than did size of high school community, the latter variable's total effect was greater.

The Future of Research in Physician Career Choice

When the Longitudinal Study began, data collection and establishment of a database was a major effort. Questionnaires had to be devised and printed; students had to be assembled as a group for administration of instruments or they had to be mailed out for incoming students; responses on paper answer sheets had to be punched on computer cards; large boxes of such cards had to be lugged to a computer center; data analyses had to be run in relatively small batches while contending with slip-ups by the card-reader; reports had to be transferred from huge computer print-outs to typed 8.5 by11 paper; etc. In the present day that can all be handled with ease. Questionnaires can be set up on Google Forms, respondents can log on to the questionnaires using their computers or cell phones, enter their responses and have them automatically show up on a spreadsheet or database far away. Numbers of respondents or numbers of items present no technical barriers and analyses can be quickly carried out on a desktop computer. Thus, the technical obstacles to carrying out a large scale study no longer exist.

Problems that continue to exist include maintaining the continuity and integrity of a research group, obtaining and maintaining funding, and obtaining cooperation of respondents while not overloading them with requests for participation. Incorporating a way for students to easily obtain information from the study in order to help them make their career decisions might help in the latter regard. Considering the complexity of the medical care system and its potential for rapid change, any future research should probably be considered as a *continuous* effort rather than a long-term project.

It is doubtful that a single comprehensive database could be developed to handle all the different information needs of the various interested parties at the present time, given the competing power centers in medicine, politics and government, but researchers and data collectors might be encouraged to share their different "parts of the elephant" to their mutual benefit.

It probably would be best for a consortium or alliance of medical schools to be involved in coordinated research in order to increase the ability to generalize results, allow rapid accumulation of data, generate new ideas through synergism, and permit inclusion of institutional variables (including curricular variables). Subgroups of schools might want to focus on different aspects of career development and have a common set of measures. However, in all participating schools, data should be collected on a wide range of career disposition variables, such as in the Career Rating and Preference Inventory. Use of bipolar approach-avoidance scales rather than reliance on categorical "choices" for career variables allows observation of fluctuations in the strength of career dispositions over time and as a result of different experiences and makes it possible to use more powerful statistical techniques for analysis. Work on development of mid level concepts suitable for a numerical model of physician career dispositions and eventual choice should continue. If such a model could be assembled, it would allow prediction of changes in the output of different kinds of physicians with changes in selection procedures, curricular changes, optional funding patterns and as yet unknown influences.

Medical Education and Health Care Planning

Finally, I close this volume by reiterating the words of my esteemed colleague of 50 years, John R. Graham, MD in his anticipation of trends for the future in medical education and health care planning, as outlined in his Preface:

- The collective impact of medical schools working in new alliances will add efficiency to medical education and health care delivery in the immediate and long-term use of our limited resources

- Shifting needs in our changing world will require educators and clinicians in all settings to work in a new level of trust with colleagues around the globe

- The greater good for mankind searching for peace, health, education, and living together in new relationships will stimulate creative consortia and shared programming to improve global survival

- Longitudinal research methodology studying change over longer-term periods will be essential to responsive, reasonable, and rational interventions to maintain a careful balance between needs of the population and constraints on use of precious resources available to all countries and peoples

- Should peace and cessation of violence be seen as a public health issue, imagine the advances we could make in the next fifty years for global survival, balance, meaning, and satisfaction

◆ Scientific data for decision making in education and life sciences will become an international necessity

11 REFERENCES

1. Carnegie Commission on Higher Education, A Special Report and Recommendations. Higher Education and the Nation's Health: Policies for Medical and Dental Education. New York: McGraw-Hill Book Company, 1970.

2. Reuben A. Kessel, The A.M.A. and the Supply of Physicians, 35 *Law and Contemporary Problems* 267-283 (Spring 1970). https://scholarship.law.duke.edu/lcp/vol35/iss2/4

3. Rabinowitz, HK, Recruitment, Retention, and Follow-up of Graduates of a Program to Increase the Number of Family Physicians in Rural and Underserved Areas. N Engl J Med 1993; 328:934-939. DOI: 10.1056/NEJM199304013281307

4. Sammons, James H. Health Manpower in the Medical Marketplace, https://www.healthaffairs.org/doi/full/10.1377/hlthaff.1.4.20

5. Peterson, SE and Rodin, AE, GMENAC report on U.S. physician manpower policies: recommendations and reactions. Health Policy Educ. 1983 Apr;3(4):337-49.

6. Kennedy, V. C., Linder, S. H., & Spears, W. (1987). Estimating the Impact of State Manpower Policy: A Case Study of Reducing Medical School Enrollments. *Journal of Health Politics, Policy and Law, 12* (2), 299-311. https://corescholar.libraries.wright.edu/comhth/270. **DOI** 10.1215/03616878-12-2-299

7. State-Level Projections of Supply and Demand for Primary Care Practitioners: 2013-2025 November 2016 .U.S. Department of Health and Human Services Health Resources and Services Administration Bureau of Health Workforce National Center for Health Workforce Analysis https://bhw.hrsa.gov/sites/default/files/bhw/health-workforce-analysis/research/projections/primary-care-state-projections2013-2025.pdf

8. 2018 Update:The Complexities of Physician Supply and Demand: Projections from 2016 to 2030 Final Report. Prepared for: Association of American Medical Colleges Submitted by: IHS Markit Ltd March 2018 https://aamc-

black.global.ssl.fastly.net/production/media/filer_public/bc/a9/bca9725e-3507-4e35-87e3-d71a68717d06/aamc_2018_workforce_projections_update_april_11_2018.pdf

9. The National Council Medical Director Institute. The Psychiatric Shortage: Causes and Solutions. March 28, 2017. https://www.thenationalcouncil.org/wp-content/uploads/2017/03/Psychiatric-Shortage_National-Council-.pdf

10. Mitchell, Wayne D. Medical Student Career Choice: A Conceptualization, Social Science and Medicine, 9, 1975, 641-653.

11. Jeffe, DB, Whelan, AJ, and Andriole, DA. Primary Care Specialty Choices of United States Medical Graduates, 1997–2006 . *Acad Med.* 2010; 85:947–958.

12. Muscatello, MRA, Bruno, A, Genovese, G, Gallo, G, Zoccali, RA, Battaglia, F. Personality traits predict a medical student preference to pursue a career in surgery. *Education for Health* Volume 30, Issue 3 (September-December 2017), 211-214.

13. Bowman, RC. Five periods of Health Policy and Physician Career Choice. October 30, 2006. http://www.ruralmedicaleducation.org/five_periods_of_health_policy.htm

14. Otis, G, Graham, J, and Thacher, L., Typological analysis of U. S. medical schools. *Journal of Medical Education*, 1975 (Apr), Vol. 50, 328-338.

15. Quenk, N. A retrospective study of past participants in AMSA Foundation programs. A report to The Bureau of Health Manpower, DHEW, Contract No. 231-75-0606, 1976.

16. Borges, NJ, and Savickas, ML. Personality and Medical Specialty Choice: A Literature Review and Integration. *Journal of Career Assessment*, Vol. 10 No. 3, August 2002 362–380.

17. Otis, G, Quenk, N, Weiss, J., Albert, M., Mitchell, W., and Richardson, C., *Medical Specialty Selection: A Review.* Washington: DHEW Publication No. (HRA) 75-8, May, 1974.

18. Zeldow PB, Preston RC, Daugherty SR. The decision to enter a medical specialty: timing and stability. *Med Educ.* 1992;26(4):327–32. https://doi.org/10.1111/j.1365-2923.1992.tb00177.x

19. Kassebaum DG, Szenas PL. Medical students' career indecision and specialty rejection: roads not taken. *Acad Med.* 1995;70(10):937–43.

20. Scott I, Gowans M, Wright B and Brenneis F. Stability of medical student career interest: a prospective study. *Acad Med.* 2012;87(9):1260–7

21. Compton MT, Frank E, Elon L, Carrera J. Changes in U.S. medical students' specialty interests over the course of medical school. *J Gen Intern Med.* 2008;23(7):1095–100.

22. Goldacre, MJ, Laxton, L, and Lambert, TW. Medical graduates' early career choices of specialty and their eventual specialty destinations: UK prospective cohort studies. *BMJ* 2010;340:c3199. doi:10.1136/bmj.c3199.

23. Jones,MD,Yamashita, T, Ross, RG and Gong, J. Positive predictive value of medical student

specialty choices. *BMC Medical Education* (2018) 18:33 https://doi.org/10.1186/s12909-018-1138-x

24. *AAMC 2012 Physician Specialty Data Book*, Table 5, column 2, "Active US M.D.s", (https://www.aamc.org/download/313228/data/2012physicianspecialtydatabook.pdf).

25. Myers, I. B., *The Myers-Briggs Type Indicator*, Manual, (Princeton, N. J.: Educational Testing Service, 1962).

26. Myers, IB, McCaulley, MH, Quenk, N, and Hammer, AL. *MBTI Manual: A guide to the development and use of the Myers-Briggs Type Indicator*, Third Edition. Consulting Psychologists Press: Palo Alto, CA, 1998.

27. Cattell, R. B., Eber H. and Tatsuoka, M., *Handbook for the Sixteen Personality Factor Questionnaire* (Champaign, Ill.:Institute for Personality and Ability Testing,1970).

28. Cattell, R. B., Cattell, A. K., & Cattell, H. E. (1993). *Sixteen Personality Factor Questionnaire* (5th ed.). Champaign, IL: Institute for Personality and Ability Testing.

29. Otis, G. *Random Sampler* (Database program for conducting Monte Carlo analyses of continuous-categorical data and categorical data between groups, with support routines), Copyright Gerald D. Otis, 1996 – 2001.

30. Otis, G. *SRTT for the MBTI* (Program to compute selection ratio type tables for the Myers-Briggs Type Indicator using observed and expected numbers of cases), Copyright Gerald D. Otis, 2017.

31. McCaulley, M. H. (1978). Application of the Myers-Briggs Type Indicator to medicine and other health professions. Monograph I, Contract No. 231-76-0051, Health Resources Administration, DHEW. Gainesville, FL: Center for Applications of Psychological Type.

32. Gerald P. Macdaid, Mary H. McCaulley and Richard I. Kainz. *Myers-Briggs Type Indicator Atlas of Type Tables*. Center for Applications of Psychological Type, Gainesville, FL, 1991. ISBN: 9780935652130.

33. Myers, IB, and Davis, JA. Relation of medical students' psychological type to their specialties twelve years later: A paper presented at the 1964 annual meeting of the American Psychological Association, Los Angeles, CA, September 4-9, 1964. Educational Testing Service, Princeton, New Jersey, December, 1964.

34. Borges, NJ, and Savickas, ML. Personality and medical specialty choice, op. cit.

35. Borges, N. J., & Osmon, W. R. (2001). Personality and medical specialty choice: Technique orientation versus people orientation. *Journal of Vocational Behavior*, 58, 22-35.

36. Taber, BJ, Hartung, PJ and Borges, NJ. Personality and values as predictors of medical specialty choice. *Journal of Vocational Behavior*, April 2011, 78(2):202-209.Available from: https://www.researchgate.net/publication/232359711_Personality_and_values_as_predictors_of_medical_specialty_choice [accessed Jul 20 2018].

37. Myers, IB, and Davis, JA. Relation of medical students' psychological type to their specialties

twelve years later, op. cit.

38. Taylor, A. D., Clark, C., & Sinclair, A. E. (1990). Personality types of family practice residents in the 1980's. *Academic Medicine*, 65, 216-218.

39. Stilwell, N. A., Wallick, M. M., Thal, S. E., & Burleson, J. A. (2000). Myers-Briggs type and medical specialty choice: A new look at an old question. *Teaching and Learning in Medicine*, 12(1), 14-20.

40. Taber et al. Personality and values as predictors of medical specialty choice. op. cit.

41. Chong Yang, George Richard, Martin Durkin. The association between Myers-Briggs Type Indicator and Psychiatry as the specialty choice. *International Journal of Medical Education*. 2016;7:48-51

42. Friedman, C. P., & Slatt, L. M. (1988). New results relating the Myers-Briggs Type Indicator and medical specialty choice. *Journal of Medical Education*, 63, 325-327.

43. Jeffe, et al. Primary Care Specialty Choices of United States Medical Graduates, op. cit.

44. Kassebaum DG, Szenas PL. Medical students' career indecision and specialty rejection: roads not taken. *Acad Med*. 1995;70(10):937–43.

45. Jones,MD,Yamashita, T, Ross, RG and Gong, J. Positive predictive value of medical student specialty choices. *BMC Medical Education* (2018) 18:33 https://doi.org/10.1186/s12909-018-1138-x

46. Looney, SW, Blondell, RD, Gogel, JR and Pentecost, MW. Which medical school applicants will become generalists or rural-based physicians? *J Ky Med Assoc*. 1998;96(5):189–93.

47. Scott I, Gowans M, Wright B and Brenneis F. Stability of medical student career interest: a prospective study. *Acad Med*. 2012;87(9):1260–7

48. Compton MT, Frank E, Elon L, Carrera J. Changes in U.S. medical students' specialty interests over the course of medical school. *J Gen Intern Med*. 2008;23(7):1095–100.

49. Otis, GD, Mosier, W, Smith, SW and Chesson, A. SAMA – MECO: A student preceptorship program and determinants of its perceived success (1974). Report pursuant to Contract No. HSM 110-72-388 with the Health Services Administration, DHEW.

50. Zimny, C. and Thale, T., "Specialty Choice and Attitudes towards Medical Specialties," *Social Science and Medicine*, 4 (1970) 257-264.

51. Bruhn, J. G. and Parsons, O. A., "Attitudes toward Medical Specialties: Two Follow-up Studies," *J. Med. Ed.*, 40 (1965) 273-280.

52. Kane, CK. Updated Data on Physician Practice Arrangements: Physician Ownership Drops Below 50 Percent. *AMA Economic and Health Policy Research*, May 2017. https://www.ama-assn.org/sites/default/files/media-browser/public/health-policy/PRP-2016-physician-benchmark-survey.pdf

53. Kletke, PR, Emmons, DW and Gillis, KD. Current trends in physician' practice arrangements: from owners to employees. *JAMA*, 1996;276(7):555-560.

https://jamanetwork.com/journals/jama/article-abstract/406731.

54. Kash, B and Tan, D. Physician group practice trends: A comprehensive review. *J Hospital and Medical Management*, Mar. 21, 2016. http://hospital-medical-management.imedpub.com/physician-group-practice-trends-a-comprehensive-review.php?aid=9343

55. Rappleye, E. 15 key findings on physician practice arrangements. *Becker's Hospital Review*, July 08, 2015. https://www.beckershospitalreview.com/hospital-physician-relationships/15-key-findings-on-physician-practice-arrangements.html

56. Medicus News Post. 2017 Physician Practice Preference and Relocation Survey - The Medicus Firm Releases 14th Annual Report. July 5, 2017. https://www.themedicusfirm.com/news/2017-physician-practice-preference-and-relocation-survey---the-medicus-firm-releases-14th-annual-report.

57. Dyrda, L. 112 statistics on physicians under 45 years old — practice setting, finances, future plans & more. *Becker's Hospital Review*, November 2, 2016. https://www.beckershospitalreview.com/hospital-physician-relationships/112-statistics-on-physicians-under-45-years-old-practice-setting-finances-future-plans-more.html

58. Ubokudom, SE. The association between the organization of medical practice and primary care physician attitudes and practice orientations. *Social Science and Medicine*, Vol. 46(1), January 1998, 59-71.

59. Wolinsky, FD. Why physicians choose different types of practice settings. *Health Services Research* 17:4 (Winter 1982), 399-419.

60. Quenk, N and Albert, M. A taxonomy of physician work settings. Study report 2 to the Bureau of Health Resources Development, Health Resource Administration, Contract No. 1-MI-24197, 1975.

61. Quenk, N. Sources of physician satisfaction. A report to the Bureau of Health Manpower, Health Resources Administration. Contract No. 1-MI-24197, 1975.

62. Rivo, ML, and Kindig, DA. A Report Card on the Physician Work Force in the United States. *N Engl J Med* 1996; 334:892-896. https://www.nejm.org/doi/full/10.1056/NEJM199604043341405.

63. Bible, BL. Physicians' views of medical practice in non-metropolitan communities, *Public Health Reports* 85:11, 1970.

64. Sax, E. *Distribution of Health Manpower: An annotated bibliography*. National Health Council, NY, April 1973.

65. Rabinowitz, HK and Paynter, NP. The rural vs urban practice decision. *AMA*. 2002;287(1):113. doi:10.1001/jama.287.1.113-JMS0102-7-1.

66. Otis, G, The effects of preceptorship location on medical students' dispositions toward small town practice, 1976. Unpublished report.

67. Henry JA, Edwards BJ, Crotty B. Why do medical graduates choose rural careers? *Rural Remote Health*. 2009 Jan-Mar;9(1):1083. Epub 2009 Feb 28. http://www.ncbi.nlm.nih.gov/pubmed/19257797.

68. Elam, CL, Rosenbaum, ME and Johnson, MMS. Geographic origin and its impact on practice location in Kentucky. *J Ky Med Assoc.* 1996;94(October):446–450.

69. Looney, SW, Blondell, RD, Gogel, JR and Pentecost, MW. Which medical school applicants will become generalists or rural-based physicians? *J Ky Med Assoc.* 1998;96(5):189–93.

70. Bowman, RC. Rural workforce past, present and future. Undated. http://www.ruralmedicaleducation.org/basichealthaccess/Rural_Born_Changes.htm

71. Bowman, RC. By the numbers: rural doctors and rural economies. http://www.ruralmedicaleducation.org/fedstloc/by_the_numbers.htm

72. Bowman, RC. They really do go. *Rural and Remote Health* 2008; 8: 1035. Available: www.rrh.org.au/journal/article/1035.

73. Bowman, RC. Why doctor's don't go where they're needed. http://www.ruralmedicaleducation.org/why_docs_dont.htm.

74. Bowman, RC. Physician workforce studies. http://www.ruralmedicaleducation.org/physician_workforce_studies.htm

75. AAFP. Rural Practice, Keeping Physicians In (Position Paper). Undated. https://www.aafp.org/about/policies/all/rural-practice-paper.html

76. Quenk, N.and Albert, M. *A Taxonomy of Physician Work Settings.* Study report #2 to Bureau of Health Resources Development. Health Resource Administration Contract No. 1-MI-24197, 1975.

77. Tryon, P.C. and Bailey. D.L *Cluster Analysis*, New York; McGraw-Hill Publishers. 1970.

78. Quenk, N. and Heffron, W. Types of Family Practice Teachers· and Residents: A Comparative Study, *Journal of Family Practice*, 1975, Vol. 2, No. 3, 195-200.

79. Mccaulley M: *The Myers-Briggs Type Indicator in Medical Education*. Washington, DC. AAMC, 1974.

80. Myers IB, Davis, JA: Relation of medical students' psychological type to their specialties twelve years later. *Research Memorandum, RM-6415*, Priniceton , NJ, Educational Testing Service, 1965.

81. Myers, I.B. and MacCaulley, M.H. Relevance of Type to Medical Education. Unpublished manuscript, March 1973.

82. Arasteh, J.D.: Factors Influencing Practice Location of Professional Health Manpower: A Review of the Literature. *DHEW. Publication No. (HRA) 75-3*, 1974.

83. Presser, C.J.: Factors affecting the geographic distribution of physicians. *J. Legal Medicine*

3:16, 1975

84. Sax, E.: *Distribution of Health Manpower: An Annotated Bibliography*. National Health Council, New York, April, 1973.

85. *Review of Incentive Programs Promoting Practice in Under-served Areas*. National Health Council, New York, February, 1976

86. Eisenberg, B.S., and Cantwell, J.R.: Policies to influence the spatial distribution of physicians: a conceptual review of selected programs and empirical evidence. *Med. Care* 14:455, 1976.

87. *A Directory of Preceptorship Programs in the Health Professions*. National Health Council, New York, August, 1975

88. Steinwald, B., and Steinwald, C.: The effect of preceptorship and rural training programs on physicians' practice location decisions. *Med. Care* 13:223, 1975.

89. Bible, B.L.: Physicians' views of medical practice in non-metropolitan communities. *Public Health Reports* 85: 11, 1970.

90. Sivertson, S.E., and Stone, H.L.: Is the preceptorship an anachronism, *JAMA* 221:590, 1972.

91. Blalock, H.M. (Ed.): *Causal Models in the Social Sciences.* New York, Aldine-Atherton, 1971

92. Heise, D.R.: Problems in path analysis and causal inference. In E.F. Borgatta, Ed., *Sociological Methodology*. San Francisco, Jossey Bass, 1969.

93. Wright, S.: Path coefficients and path regressions: alternative or complimentary concepts.. *Biometrics* 16:189, 1960.

Gerald Otis and Naomi Quenk

Appendix

Gerald D. Otis

This chapter describes the process and results of selecting and developing assessment devices to be used in the Longitudinal Study. Instruments included two personality questionnaires, an index of certain aspects of physician ideology, a student-faculty role questionnaire, an instrument to assess various kinds of background characteristics, an assessment of a range of career inclinations, a clerkship socialization intensity questionnaire, an internship-residency inventory, and a physician work-setting instrument. Averages at different time periods are shown for the scales of the Physician Ideology Questionnaire and selected items on the Career Rating and Preference Questionnaire. Averages during different medical school years for different psychological types are presented for selected scales of the Student-Faculty Role Questionnaire. Items for each of the questionnaires developed by the Longitudinal Study are presented in full following the general descriptions.

Personality Scales

We believed from the beginning that personality processes must play a significant role in making decisions about future careers as well as differing orientation toward various aspects of medicine and the early research on medical career choice supported that assumption. At the time, the two most used non-pathology oriented personality questionnaires were the *Myers-Briggs Type Indicator* (MBTI) developed by Katherine Briggs and Isabel Briggs Myers and the *16 Personality Factor Questionnaire (16PF)* developed by Raymond B. Cattell and colleagues. We decided to include both of those inventories, to be administered as early as possible in the student's process of medical education.

The MBTI was based on Carl Jung's theory of Psychological Types and claimed to measure a person's status on two orientations toward energy (Introversion and Extraversion), two ways of taking in information (Sensing and Intuition) and two methods of coming to conclusions (Thinking and Feeling). Jung combined a person's energy orientation with the other four mental processes to define eight mental functions: Introverted Sensing, Introverted Intuition, Introverted Thinking, Introverted Feeling and the four

Extraverted versions of those processes. Isabel Myers added on a fourth bi-polar contrast : Judging and Perceiving, in order to identify which of the processes were either auxiliary or dominant in a particular personality. The result was a scheme that identified 16 different types of personality, designated by their initial letters except for Intuition which was designated by N. Thus, a person might be identified as an INTP where Introverted Thinking is the dominant function and Extraverted Intuition is the auxiliary function. It should be remembered that the basic distinctions are really bi-polar contrasts rather than positions on a continuous dimension. However, a concession to dimensionality was made in that the MBTI also contains a "continuous score" that presumably measures the degree of affinity toward one side of the contrast or the other. So, in fact, there are several indexes that can be derived for an individual on the MBTI: her or his designation on the four contrasts (E-I, S-N, T-F, J-P); the four corresponding continuous scores, the individuals Psychological Type (a concatenation of 4 letters), and the person's dominant, auxiliary, tertiary and inferior functions. (More recent versions of the MBTI have added a second layer of scoring that identifies "facets" within functions, but that refinement was not available at the time this study was initiated). The four basic contrasts of the MBTI appear to correspond to four of the five factors in the widely adopted Five Factor Theory of Personality, with only a measure of anxiety being left out. However, there appear to be things that the MBTI picks up on that the Five Factor model does not (and vice versa).

The 16 PF was a more empirically constructed instrument, based on factor analyses of numerous item pools with different population samples over the many years of its construction. Cattell relied not only on questionnaire items but also used observational data and experimental data in his search for a set of dimensions that would adequately describe personality variations. Originally, he did not want to import extraneous meaning and associations into the description of the dimensions he extracted by using common language terms. Instead, he made up new terms for the opposite ends of his continua where the "meaning" was determined by the magnitude of statistical coefficients associated with the factors extracted. However, his use of terms like "Premsia," "Threctia," "Alaxia" and "Praxernia" or even use of letters like A, B, C, did not go over well with users of the instrument and everyone started attaching one or more common language terms to the ends of his dimensions of personality variation. The 16 factors were:

A. Sizothymia (reserved) vs. Affectothymia (outgoing)

B. Low Intelligence vs. High Intelligence

C. Low Ego Strength (easily upset) vs. High Ego Strength (emotionally stable)

E. Submissiveness vs. Dominance

F. Desurgency (serious) vs. Surgency (happy—go-lucky)

G. Weak Superego Strength (expedient) vs. Strong Superego Strength (conscientious)

H. Threctia (shy) vs. Parmia (socially bold)

I. Harria (tough-minded) vs. Premsia (tender—minded)

L. Alaxia (trusting) vs. Protension (suspicious)

M. Praxernia (practical) vs. Autia (imaginative)

N. Artlessness (unpretentious) vs. Shrewdness (socially aware)

O. Untroubled Adequacy (self—assured) vs. Guilt Proneness (self—reproaching)

Q1. Conservativism (respecting of traditional ideas) vs. Radicalism (experimenting)

Q2. Group Adherence (group dependence) vs. Self- Sufficiency (prefers own decisions)

Q3. Low Self-Sentiment Integration (undisciplined self-conflict) vs. High Strength of Self- Sentiment (controlled, socially precise)

Q4. Low Ergic Tension (relaxed) vs. High Ergic Tension (tense, driven)

Four second-order factors could also be derived based on combinations of scores on the primary factors: Anxiety, Extraversion vs. Introversion, Tough Poise vs. Responsive Emotionality and Independence vs. Dependence.

Physician Ideology Questionnaire

The initial items for the Physician Ideology Questionnaire (originally called the Social Role of the Ideal Physician Questionnaire) were developed by the sociologist in our Behavioral Sciences Teaching Group, Lois Dilatush, during the early years while the project was still focusing on attitude change during medical education. Items were added and deleted over the first few years and factor analyses were performed on the accumulating data set until a relatively stable factor structure was achieved. The final questionnaire is shown in Appendix A.

PIQ Factors

The factors extracted from factor analyses of items for all subjects is shown below along with item scoring weights to estimate factor scores and the average scores in standard deviation units across years in medical school.

Factor 1: Psycho-social Orientation. The degree to which the respondent considers it important for the physician to have knowledge and skill in interpersonal relations and apply that knowledge and skill to the social and emotional problems of patients.

Weighted Scoring

Total Score= $C_1 + \Sigma(I_i W_i)$ where $= C_1 = +38.20034$, $I_i =$ the item value and $W_i =$ the item weight

Items (I_i) = [2,5,6,7,28,29,30,31,32,34,37,38,39,41,43,44]

Item Weights (W_i) = [-2.17374, -2.01463, -1.92292, -1.37496, -1.19413, -1.44981, -0.65328, -1.73556, -0.92976, -0.82075, -1.10940, -1.25489, -1.07355, -0.90344, -4.22534, -0.28714]

Mean Total Score=0.00 Standard Deviation=10.9981

Percentile Equivalents

10	20	30	40	50	60	70	80	90
-14.19	-9.35	-5.83	-2.86	0	2.06	5.83	9.35	14.19

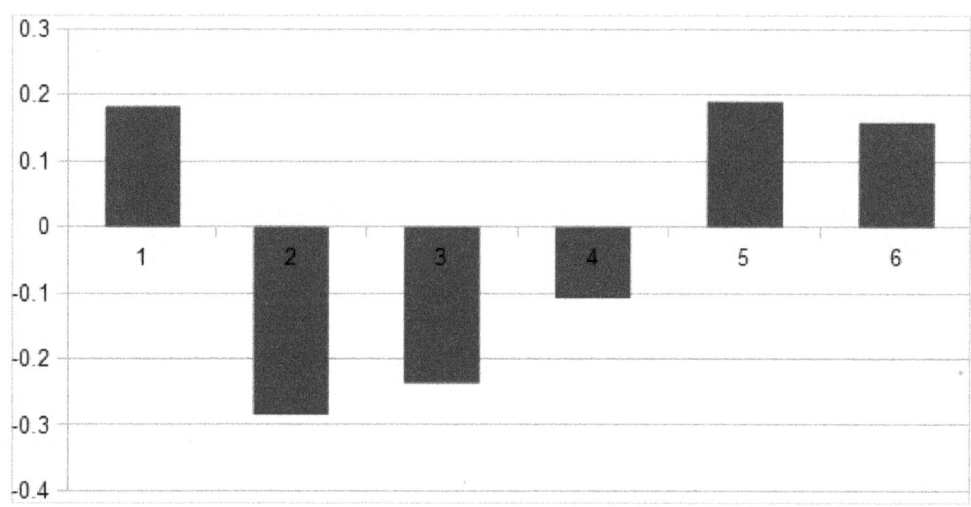

Average Value of "Psychosocial Orientation" by year from entry (1) to PG1 (6).

Factor 2: Division of Responsibility for Information Exchange. The degree to which the respondent thinks the physician (rather than the nurse) should obtain information and provide information to the patient and his/her family.

Weighted Scoring

Total Score= $C_1 + \Sigma(I_i W_i)$ where = $C_{1=}$ +12.38553, I_i= the item value and W_i= the item weight

Items (I_i) = [45,46,47,48,49,50]

Item Weights (W_i) = [-0.95072,-1.12713,-0.89984,-1.40032,-1.09038,-1.07490]

Mean Total Score=0.00 Standard Deviation= 4.2173

Percentile Equivalents

10	20	30	40	50	60	70	80	90
-5.44	-3.58	-2.24	-1.1	0	1.1	2.24	3.58	5.44

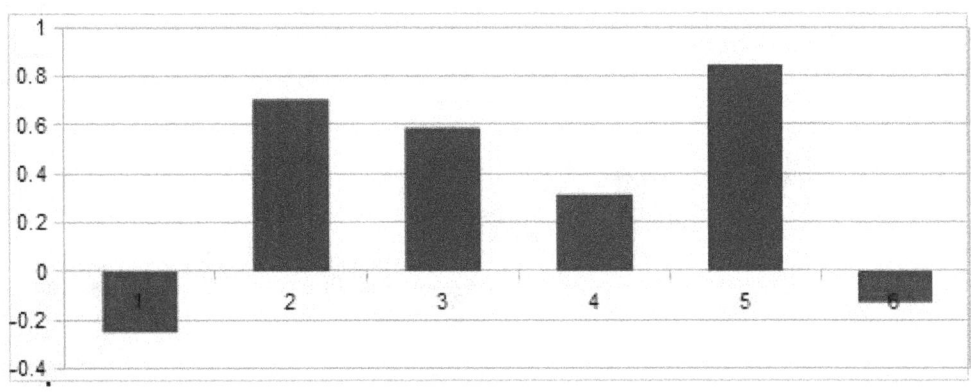

Average Value of "Division of Responsibility for Information Exchange" by year from entry to PG1.

Factor 3: Community Orientation. The degree to which the respondents considers it important that the physician be involved in health-related community activities other than patient care.

Weighted Scoring

Total Score= $C_1 + \Sigma(I_i W_i)$ where $= C_1 = +11.86415$, I_i= the item value and W_i= the item weight

Items (I_i) = [11,35,36,42]

Item Weights (W_i) = [-0.98555,-1.05607,-1.31009,-1.17977]

Mean Total Score=0.00 Standard Deviation= 4.2173

Percentile Equivalents

10	20	30	40	50	60	70	80	90
-3.66	-2.41	-1.5	-0.74	0	0.74	1.5	2.41	3.66

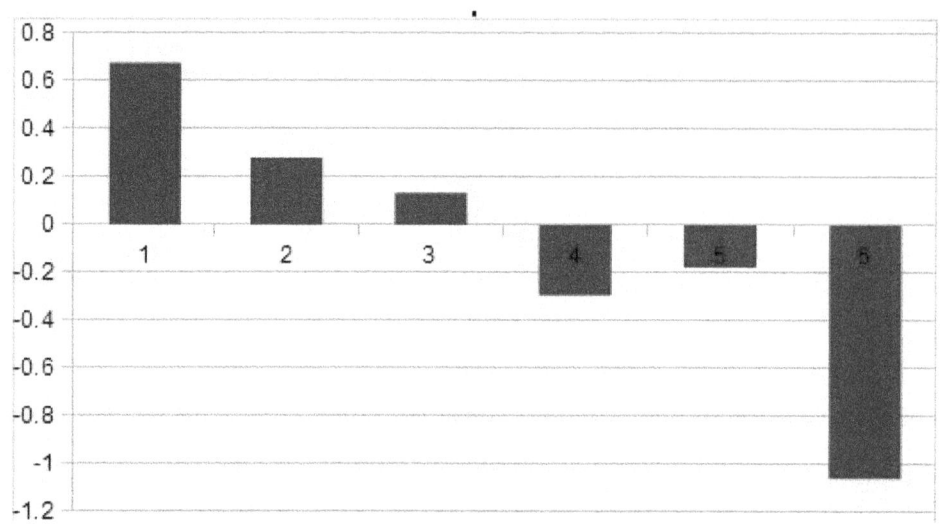

Average Value of "Community Orientation" by year from entry to PG1.

Factor 4: Biological Orientation. The degree of importance the respondent attaches to the physician's biological knowledge and skill in applying it.

Weighted Scoring

Total Score= $C_1 + \Sigma(I_i W_i)$ where = C_1 = +23.47734, I_i= the item value and W_i= the item weight

Items (I_i) = [4,8,13,18,21]

Item Weights (W_i) = [-2.65843,-2.80589,-1.48750,-1.4863,-1.31965]

Mean Total Score=0.00 Standard Deviation= 3.5010

Percentile Equivalents

10	20	30	40	50	60	70	80	90
-4.52	-2.98	-1.86	-0.91	0	0.91	1.86	2.98	4.52

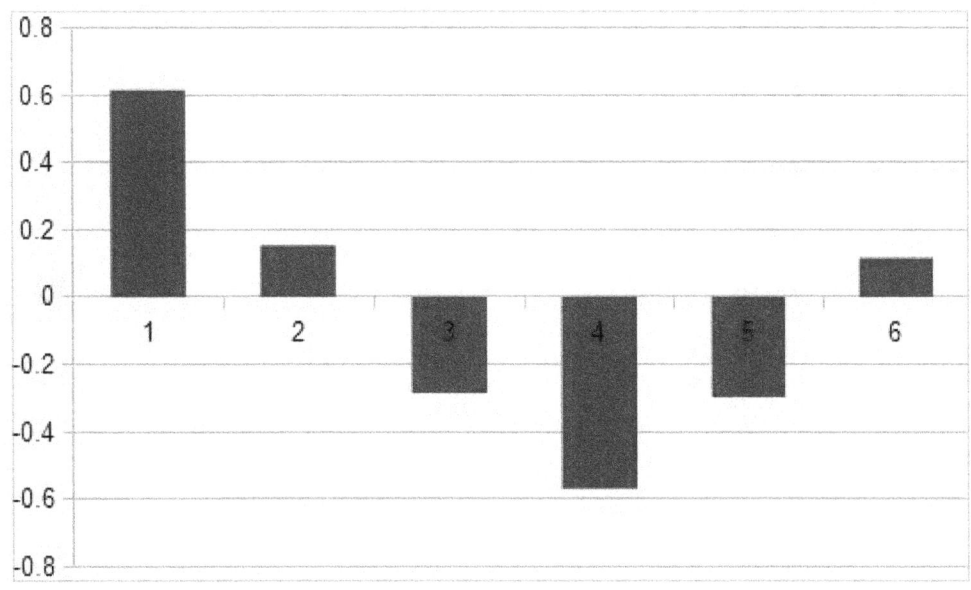

Average Value of "Biological Orientation" by year from entry (1) to PG1 (6).

Factor 5: Physician Authority. The degree to which the respondent considers it important for the physician to have control over his work setting and all aspects of patient care.

Weighted Scoring

Total Score= $C_1 + \Sigma(I_iW_i)$ where = $C_1 = +14.78421$, I_i= the item value and W_i= the item weight

Items (I_i) = [1,10,14,24,33]

Item Weights (W_i) = [-1.76079,-1.24712,-0.89969,-1.04848,-1.11407]

Mean Total Score=0.00 Standard Deviation= 3.3478

Percentile Equivalents

10	20	30	40	50	60	70	80	90
-4.32	-2.85	-1.77	-0.87	0	0.87	1.77	2.85	4.32

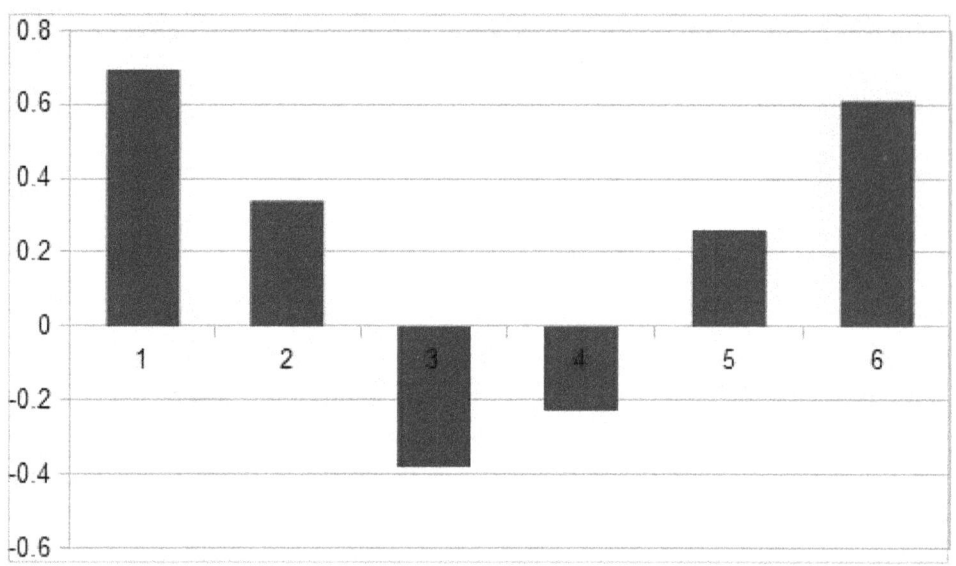

Average Value of "Physician Authority" by year from entry to PG1

Factor 6: Disease Orientation. The degree to which the respondent considers it important for the physician to focus his efforts on the treatment of biological disease rather than becoming involved in preventive and psycho-social medicine.

Weighted Scoring

Total Score= $C_1 + \Sigma(I_i W_i)$ where = $C_{1=}$ +34.57962, I_i = the item value and W_i = the item weight

Items (I_i) = [3,9,17,20,22,26,40]

Item Weights (W_i) = [-1.11979,-1.18961,-0.99359,-1.09542,-1.14361,-1.92733,-1.16230]

Mean Total Score=0.00 Standard Deviation= 4.2584

Percentile Equivalents

10	20	30	40	50	60	70	80	90
-5.49	-3.62	-2.26	-1.11	0	1.11	2.26	3.62	5.49

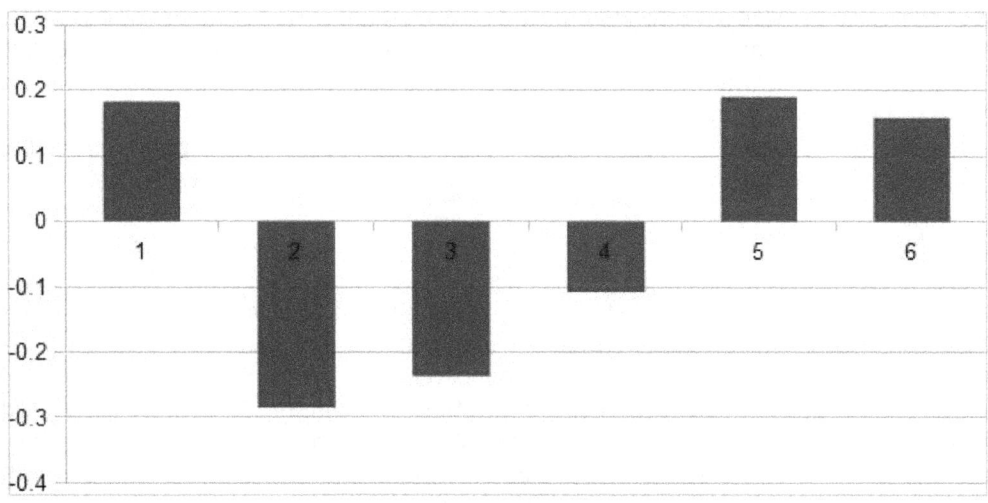

Average Value of "Disease Orientation" by year from entry (1) to PG1 (6).

Student-Faculty Role Questionnaire

The Student-Faculty Role Questionnaire was designed to assess significant dimensions of the student-faculty relationship. Following role theory, items were selected that tapped various *expectations* and *perceived enactments* of each of the participants in the relationship. Thus, each student indicated his expectations regarding how faculty members *should* behave and also how, he/she, when playing student roles, *should* behave. The respondent was also asked to indicate the degree to which her/his expectations were perceived as being met, i. e., his/her perception of the enactment of faculty and own (student) roles. Likewise, the faculty member indicated his expectations and perceived enactments regarding students and regarding himself as faculty member.

Items included in the questionnaire were samples from five domains of interaction assumed to characterize any relationship: Solidarity, Internal Instrumentality, External Relations, Goals Definition, and Division of Responsibility (cf. Tharp and Otis, 1966). Solidarity has to do with the rapport or cohesiveness of the relationship. Expectation aspects of solidarity functioning are assumed to be tapped by items like "How important is it for the ideal student-faculty relationship that faculty members should encourage students to make office visits for informal talks?" Internal Instrumentality involves how the "tasks" of the relationship should be carried out (e. g., "Faculty members should let students know what is required to meet their expectations"). External Relations has to do with relationships outside of the immediate one but involving at least one of the participants (e. g., "Faculty members should represent student views to administrative personnel"). Goals Definition concerns the specification of the aims of the relationship (e. g., Students should want to become good practitioners more than good researchers"). Division of Responsibility refers to arrangements within the other four areas; it is the differential delegation to one or another member of the responsibility and authority for originating, maintaining and terminating any activity (e. g., "Students should be involved in planning some educational sessions").

While the hypothesis of five domains of interaction provided a framework for the generation and inclusion of items in the questionnaire, they did not, by themselves, provide any specific behavioral content. The meaning, in behavioral terms, of Solidarity is quite different in a marriage relationship from what it is in a student-faculty relationship. The individual expectation and perceived enactment items provide specific content but they also provide an unwieldy mass of data. An intermediate level of description is needed. This is provided by factor analyses of the intercorrelations of item ratings which yield dimensions of individual differences along which members of the student and faculty groups vary in the strength of their expectations and perceived enactments. Besides scores for expectations and perceptions, it is possible to also generate *discrepancy score* by subtracting expectation scores from perception scores. Presumably this score would be an index of disappointment or satisfaction with the quantity of the behavior in question.

SFRQ Factors for Students

Data from the student form of the questionnaire was subjected to several different factor analyses with slightly different results for perceptions than for expectations. For consistency with role theory, it was eventually decided to score both expectation and perception portions of the questionnaire using the factor structure of the expectation section of the questionnaire. Factor scores were generated and weights were assigned to items so as to estimate factor scores directly from item scores as was done with the PIQ. However, most weights were near 1.0 (about equal weighting). Scores were then generated by simply summing the item scores for each factor. These summed scores correlated highly with the actual factor scores (r values over .90), so the weighting scheme was abandoned for simplicity.

Descriptions of the SFRQ factors are listed below along with the corresponding item numbers for the expectation and perception sections. It should be remembered that the item scales are all "inverted" such that high scores indicate a smaller quantity of the behavior in question but that all item scores are multiplied by minus one (-1.00) so that the composite score reflects a greater quantity of the attitude represented by the factor. On items listed below where there is a plus sign (+), the item value is subtracted from the cumulative sum of (item score times -1.00).

A. *Educational Goals*

1. **Psychosocial Orientation**: the value placed upon learning about psychological, social, and cultural factors in so far as they are relevant to patient care and augment clinical ability.

Expectation Items: 53, 60, 65, 66, 68, 71, 74, 75, 76, 77, 78

Perception Items: 142, 159, 145, 146, 148, 151, 154, 155, 156, 157, 158

2. **Academic Orientation**: the importance of becoming a good teacher, being theoretically oriented, developing research skills; as opposed to the importance of becoming a good clinician, being practically oriented, and gaining experience working with patients.

Expectation Items: 54, 56, 57, 58, 59, 62

Perception Items: 170, 173, 173, +171, 143

3. **Personal Development**: the importance for students to find purpose and meaning in their professional roles, to learn to understand themselves and the .complexities of the world, and to appreciate the beauty in life.

Expectation Items: 1, 65, 66, 67, 68

Perception Items: 94, 145, 146, 147, 148

B. *External Relations*

4. **Faculty Professional Activity**: the importance attributed to faculty involvement in non-teaching professional affairs - community participation, research, clinical work, medical school affairs.

Expectation Items: 81, 82, 83, 84, 85

Perception Items: 163, 164, 165, 166, 167

5. **Faculty Respectfulness**: the importance of faculty being considerate of patients during interviews and examinations, requesting their permission for procedures to be carried out, explaining procedures; also, the importance of faculty being "good examples" in their dealings with patients, being patient with students who don't understand, respecting individual student interests, etc.

Expectation Items (A): 15, 16, 17, 47

Expectation Items (B): 5, 6, 12, 15, 16, 17, 19, 33, 42, 44, 47, 75, 77

Perception Items (A): 102, 103, 104, 140

Perception Items (B): 98, 99, 108, 102, 103, 104, 105, 122, 132, 135, 140, 155, 157

C. *Internal Instrumentality*

6. **Traditional (Ideal) Student Role**: the degree to which students should really invest themselves in the work of a course, seriously consider what faculty say, be enthusiastic about learning, show interest in course material, be punctual, show academic scholarship, be orderly and productive, etc.

Expectation Items: 8, 9, 13, 14, 28, 29, 33, 34, 35, 51, 52, 69, 10

Perception Items: 110, 111, 112, 113, +117, 119, 122, 123, 124, 141, 162, 149, 152

7. **Teaching Efficiency**: the importance of faculty exciting student curiosity through teaching, specifying course requirements, accommodating to student needs, encouraging questions and discussion, giving prompt feedback, having courses well organized, being good speakers, etc.

Expectation Items: 40, 41, 43, 44, 45, 46, 49, 52

Perception Items: 130, 131, 133, 135, 136, 137, 139, 162

8. **Faculty Accommodation**: the importance of students making recommendations to faculty regarding teaching materials, methods and so on, and of faculty trying to accommodate to these suggestions.

Expectation Items: 18, 19, 20, 43

Perception Items: 114, 105, 106, 133

9. **Faculty Openness**: the importance of faculty informing students about issues of conflict within the school, revisions in school policy, what is expected of them; and of faculty allowing students free time and accommodating to student needs.

Expectation Items: 19, 20, 24, 41, 79, 80

Perception Items: 105, 106, 134, 131, 168, 169

10. **Structure**: the value placed upon faculty giving prompt feedback, specifying what is required, encouraging questions, giving recognition, evaluating by means of regular tests.

Expectation Items: 3, 41, 44, 45

Perception Items: 96, 131, 135, 136

D. Solidarity

11. **Informal Relations**: the importance of informal contacts with faculty members, e.g., informal discussions, one-to-one' talks, social affairs, office visits.

Expectation Items: 2, [25], 30, 31, 36, 37, 38, 39, 64

Perception Items: 95, [ ], 118, 120, 126, 127, 128, 129, 125

12. **Faculty Socio-emotional Role**: the degree to which faculty should go out of their way to be helpful to students, be friendly and supportive, help them to work out problems and understand themselves, etc.

Expectation Items: 1, 2, 3, 4, 5, 6, 10, 19, 20, 23, 36, 37, 38, 39, 41, 43

Perception Items: 94, 95, 96, 97, 98, 99, 100, 105, 106, 107, 126, 127, 128, 129, 131, 133

13. **Student-Faculty Camaraderie**: the importance of faculty being cheerful and humorous, getting to know students well, being included in social and unofficial affairs; and the importance of students being meticulous and persistent in their work, giving serious consideration to what faculty have to say but also making suggestions to faculty.

Expectation Items: 11, 13, 18, 31, 35, 53, 64

Perception Items: 101, 112, 114, 120, 124, 142, 125

14. **Student-Faculty Cooperation**: the value attached to students being considerate of faculty yet making suggestions to them and seeking them out for informal discussions; and of faculty being friendly and supportive, encouraging and accommodating to students and giving them' feedback concerning their performance.

Expectation Items: 8, 10, 18, 19, 30, 44, 45, 54

Perception Items: +110, 100, 114, 105, 118, 135, 136, 170

15. **Recognition**: the importance of students receiving recognition for their accomplishments, that their individuality be recognized, that they are understood and appreciated as individuals.

Expectation Items: 3, 6, 24, 31, 36, 37, 42

Perception Items: 96, 99, 134, 120, 126, 127, 122

E. *Division of Responsibility*

16. Division of Influence: the relative influence of faculty as opposed to students in preparing educational materials, deciding what's important· to learn, providing instruction, determining educational methods, choosing professional goals, specifying methods of study or learning, and in relations with administrative personnel.

Expectation Items: 86, 87, 88, 89, 90, 91, 92, 93

Perception Items: 177, 178, 179, 180, 181, 182, 183, 184

Looking at general trends in expectations and perceptions of the student-faculty relationship over time, they sometimes show general trends but mostly they obscure the differential effects of experience in medical school on different types of medical students. For example, the intellectually critical INTPs and the tenderhearted ENFPs perceive relatively the same amount of emphasis on psychosocial aspects

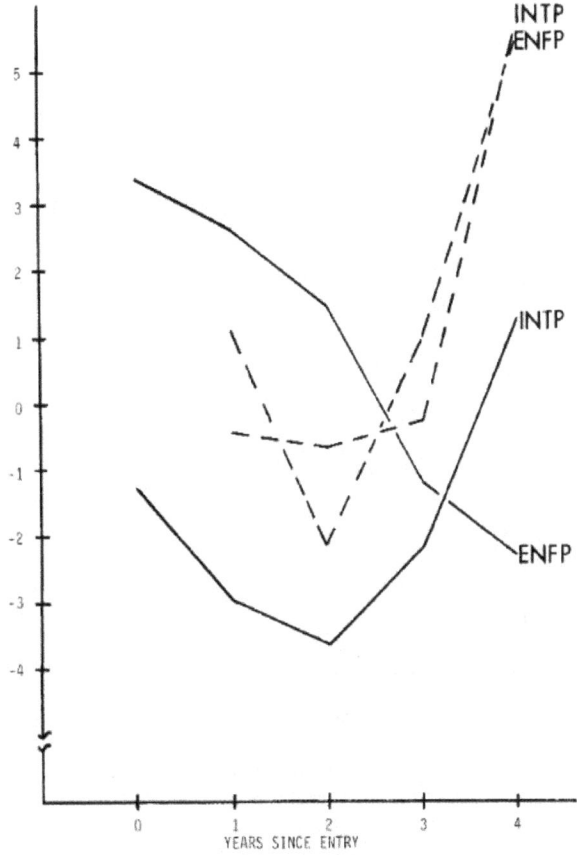

Mean scores on the Psychosocial Orientation Scales for INTP and ENFP Psychological Types. Solid lines are expectations and dashed lines are perceptions.

of medicine with that amount increasing over their years in medical school. However, their expectations (values) differ from each other at the beginning of medical school and end up with an inverted relationship to each other by the end of medical school. Both INTPs and ENFPs see a decline in the importance attributed to psychosocial aspects of medicine in their first two years but during the clinical years INTPs have a change of heart while ENFPs continue to depreciate these values.

For Faculty Respectfulness toward patients (and students), INFPs and INTJs appear to be affected in the same direction at the same time by their medical school experience with regard to both expectations and perceptions. However, perceptions are much below expectations for INFPs while the reverse is true for INTJs. Thus, one would expect INFPs to be subjectively disappointed while INTJs would be subjectively "pleasantly surprised" by what transpired.

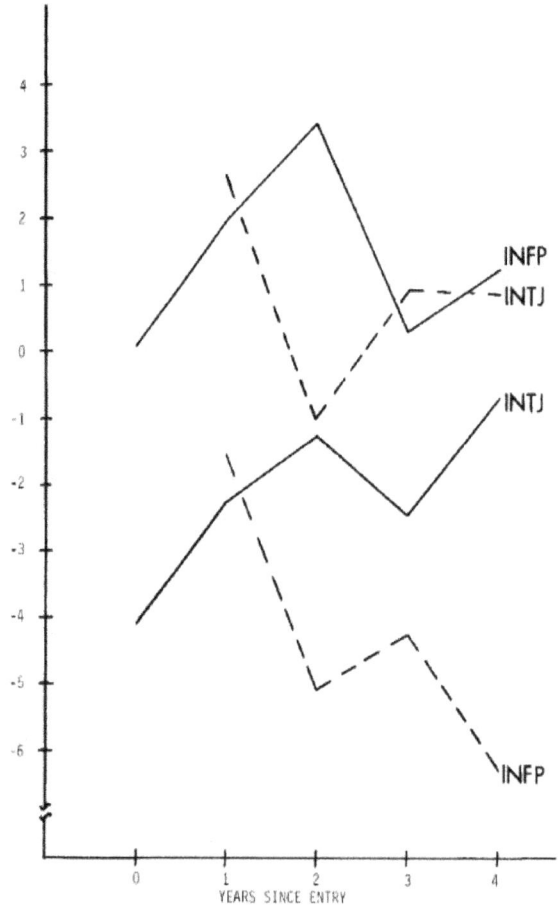

Mean scores on the Faculty Respectfulness Scales for INFPs and INTJs. Solid lines are expectations and dashed lines are perceptions.

On the Recognition Factor, INFPs are seen to consistently hold this to be of high value while ISTJs consistently hold this to be of minor value. Each gets a minor "bump" in value during the second year when they are studying for National Boards, Part I. But the two types differ radically in their perceptions of how much recognition they get, the INFPs being increasingly disappointed over the course of medical school perceive getting more recognition than expected or desired, increasingly so in the clinical years.

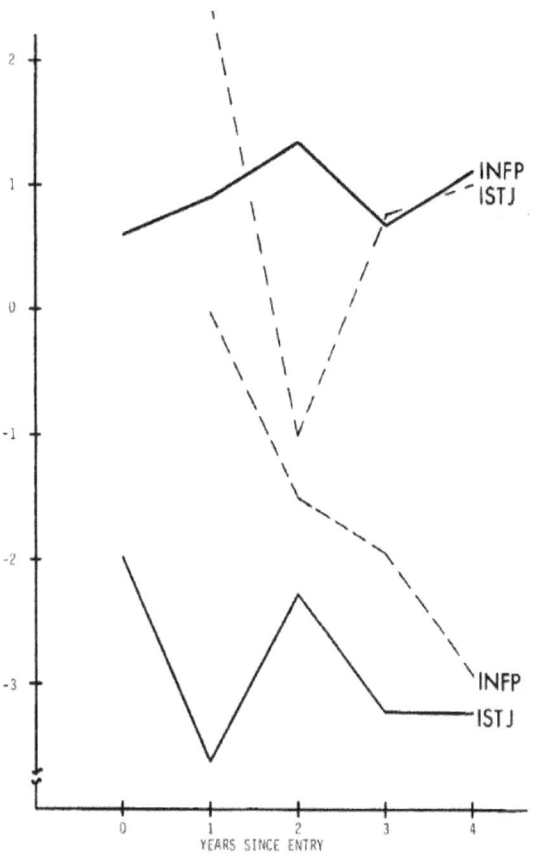

Mean scores on the Recognition Scales for INFPs and ISTJs during medical school. Solid lines are expectations and dashed lines are perceptions.

Expectations are higher for ENFJs than INFPs on the Ideal Student Role Scale with values eroding for both during the first three years but increasing by the time of graduation. Both groups perceive less emphasis in this medical school on these values during their first two years with a bump in year four. However, perceptions are lower than expectations for ENFJs while perceptions are higher than expectations for INFPs.

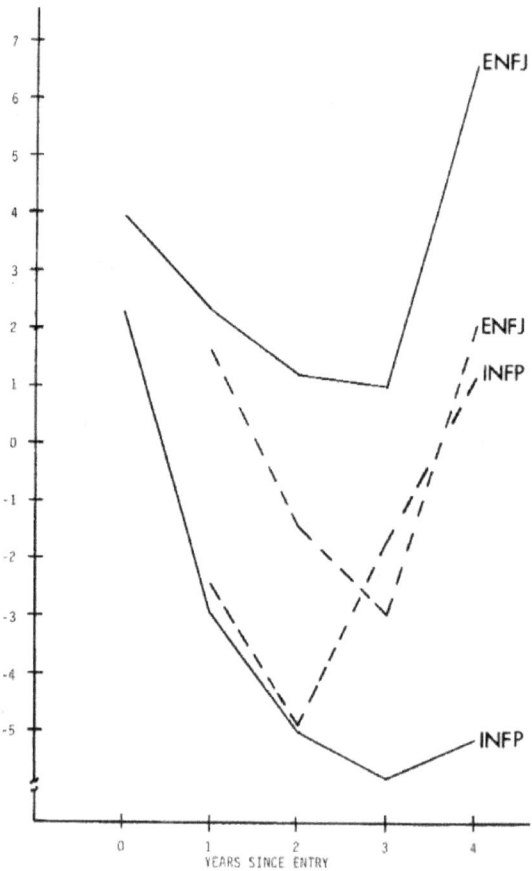

Mean scores on the Traditional/Ideal Student Role Scales for ENFJs and INFPs. Solid lines are expectations and dashed lines are perceptions

On the Personal Development Scales, INFPs have higher expectations than perceptions, ISTJs have perceptions greater than expectations and ENFPs are mixed over the course of medical school. The clinical years do not raise perceptions for INFPs while they do for both ENFPs and ISTJs. One would expect, therefore, that INFPs would become more disillusioned with the emphasis they perceive being placed on these values during medical school although they do not retreat much on the importance they ascribe to such values. While ENFPs were disillusioned during their first two years of medical school, their adherence to these values did not recover during the clinical years although their perception of the emphasis placed on such values in this medical school did show a dramatic recovery. ISTJs never placed much value on the values of Personal Development and always perceived more emphasis on such values than they desired.

Mean Scores on the Personal Development Scales during medical school for INFPs, ENFPs and ISTJs. Solid lines are expectations and dashed lines are perceptions

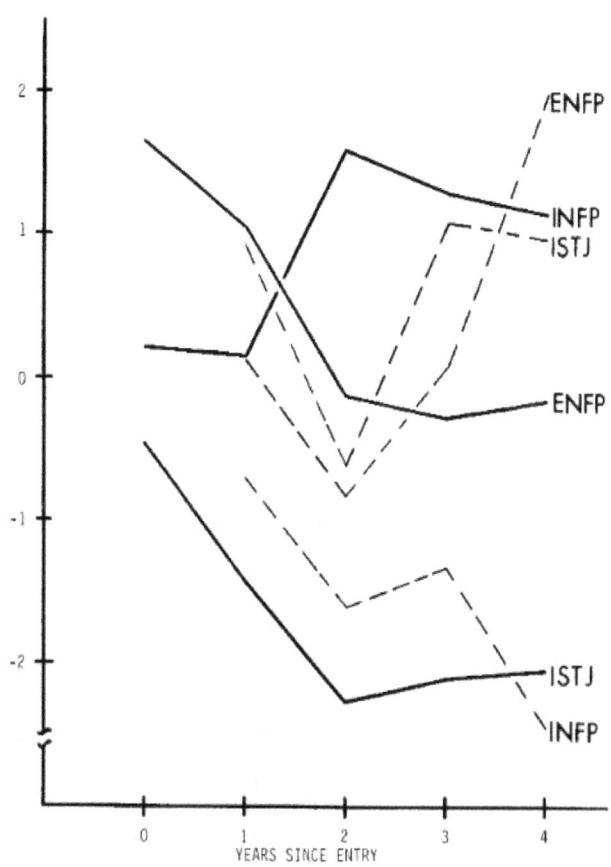

As a final example of how experience in medical school affects different types of students in different ways, we have the scores of INTPs and ENTJs on the Teaching Efficiency Scales. The independent-minded INTPs don't expect much in the way of quality teaching methods from the faculty and, except for year three, see more that they anticipated. The organized and planful ENTJs, however, expect faculty to demonstrate high standards of efficiency and are disappointed in this respect during their middle two years (although they appear to change their minds when they are seniors).

Mean scores on the Teaching Efficiency Scales for INTPs and ENTJs. Solid lines are expectations and dashed lines are perceptions

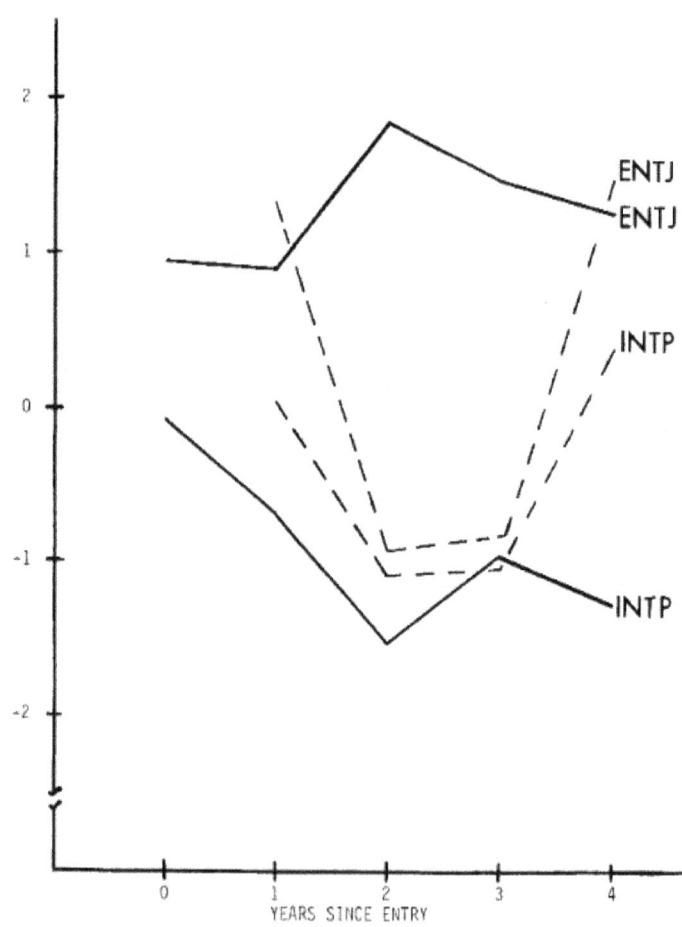

Although the SFRQ showed a lot of promise for explicating the complexities of how medical school experiences differentially affects different types of medical students, the project was terminated before that promise was fully realized. Analyses that were completed showed that faculty from different departments held different SFRQ values and saw things differently and that, surprisingly, scores on its value scales at the time of entry to medical school were significantly associated with the selection of different specialties, work settings and practice communities of different sizes.

Clerkship Socialization Intensity Questionnaire

The Clerkship Socialization Intensity Questionnaire was developed to be included as part of the mathematical modeling effort described below. Items were developed on the basis of Rue Bucher's work in professional socialization. A score was developed for each clerkship as a vector variable, i. e., as an array of weighted numbers representing various aspects of the clerkship experience. We called the variable a "clerkship socialization intensity vector" and considered it to be an index of the perceived "recruitment" efforts of the clerkship experience for each clerkship.

Career Rating and Preference Inventory

The Career Rating and Preference Inventory (fondly referred to as the CRAPI by the research staff) was gradually developed over the years to assess the fate and perturbations of various career preferences as students traversed medical school, mastered postgraduate education and eventually entered practice. We wanted to be able to track the strength of student inclinations toward different specialties, work setting and communities. We also wanted to assess how much they debated within themselves various "considerations" such as work-setting characteristics, work activities, family matters, community characteristics in the process of thinking about their careers. And we wanted to know when these inclinations stabilized and when the students stopped information processing about the particular area. Eventually, we wanted to be able to relate these measures to personality type, medical school experiences and eventual career decisions. The questionnaire is presented below:

Some illustrative charts of mean strength of preferences from the time of medical school entry to ten years later using semi-longitudinal data are shown below.

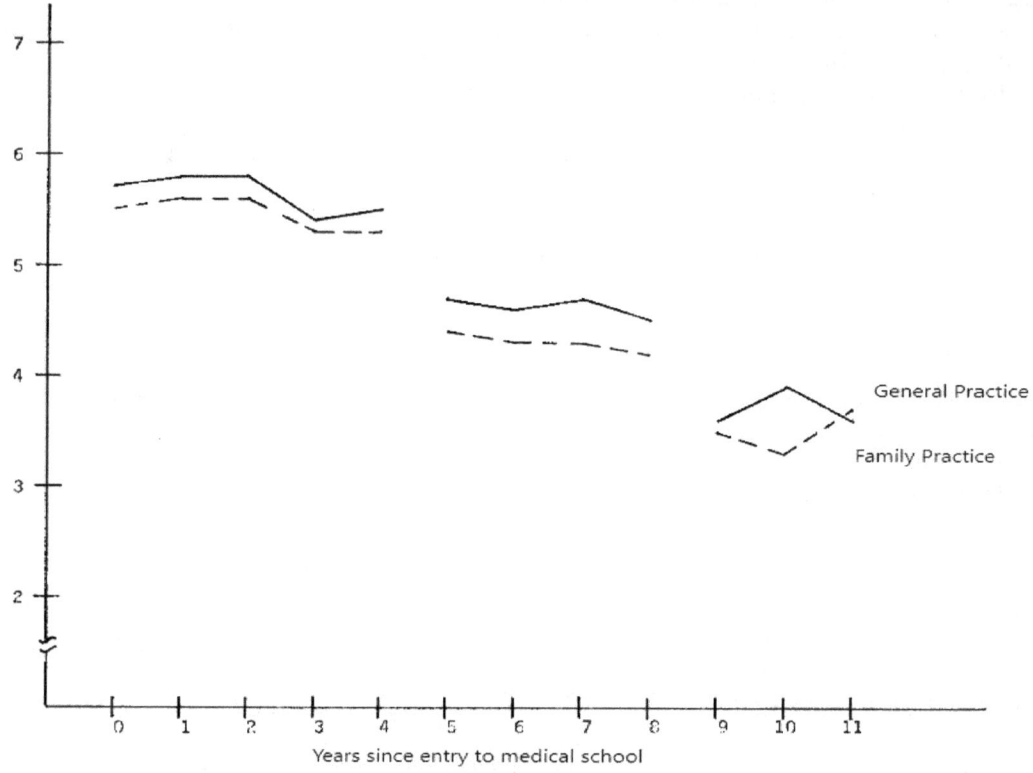

Specialty Preferences: General and Family Practice. Continuous segments use same cases.

Physician Career Choice and Satisfaction

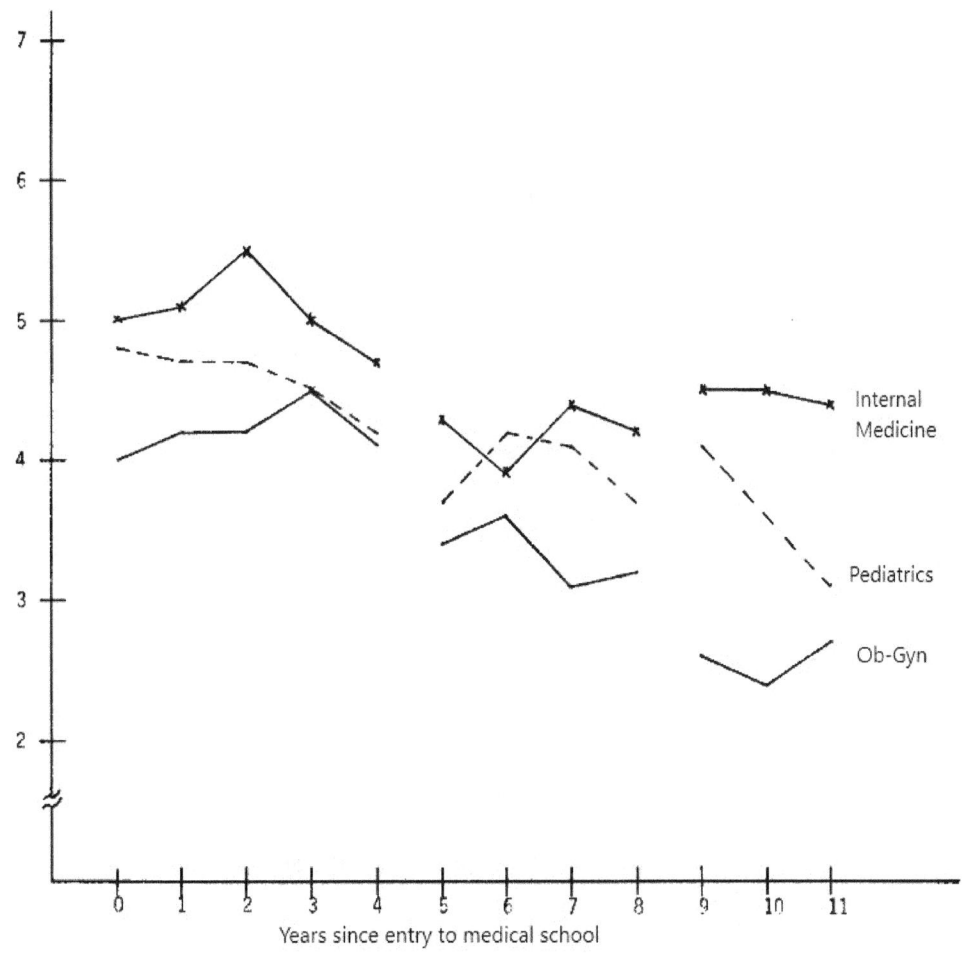

Specialty Preferences: Internal Medicine, Pediatrics and Ob-Gyn.

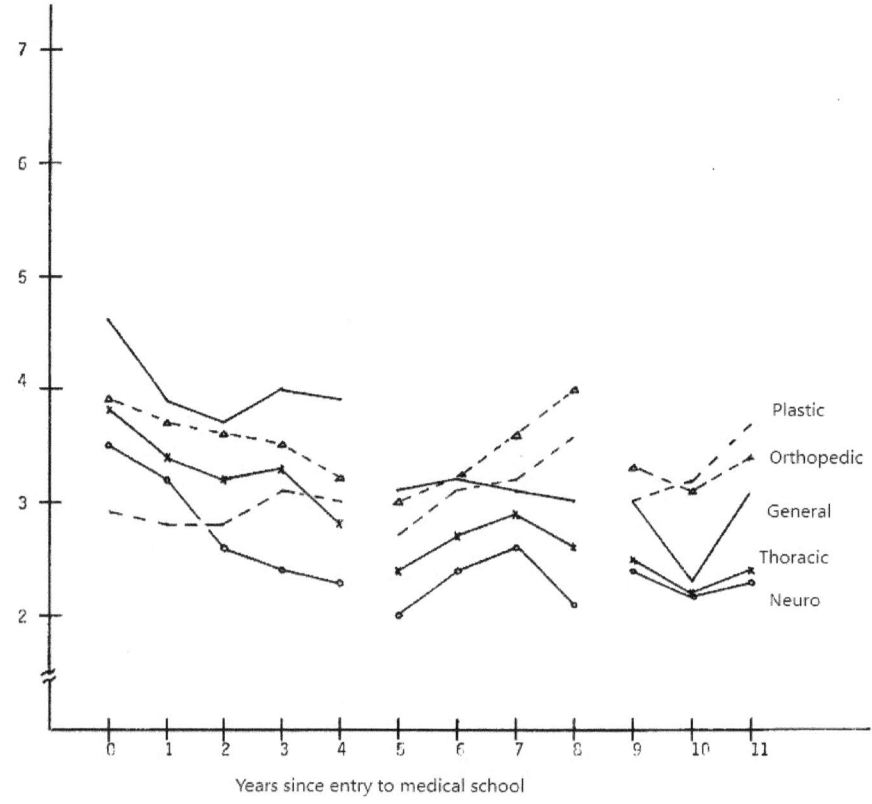

Specialty Preferences: Surgery (General and Sub-specialties).

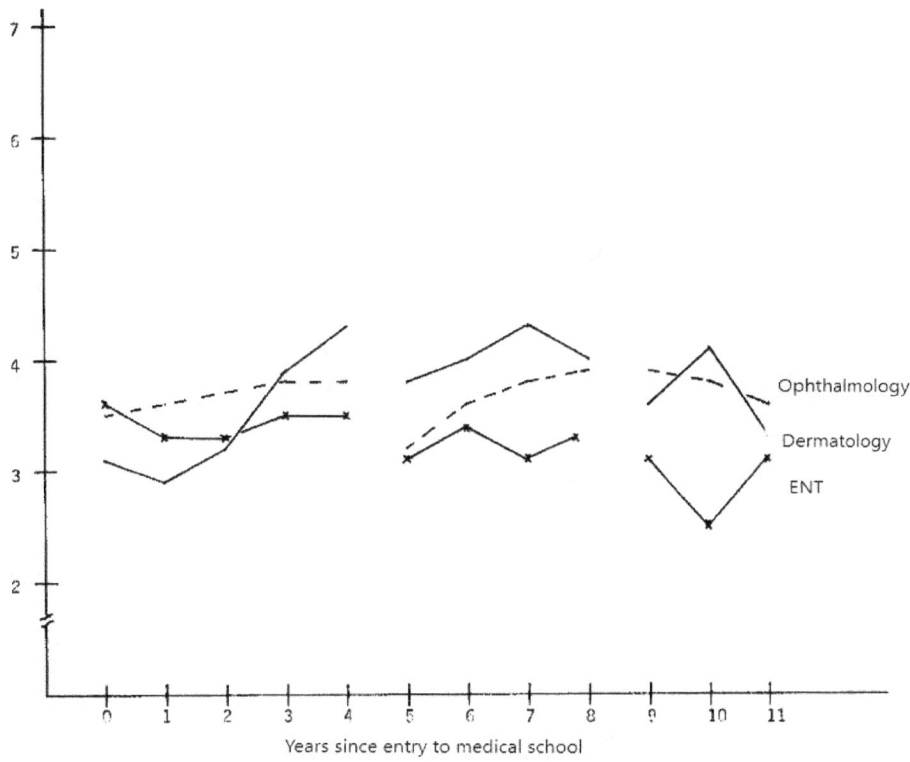

Specialty Preferences: Ophthalmology, Dermatology and ENT

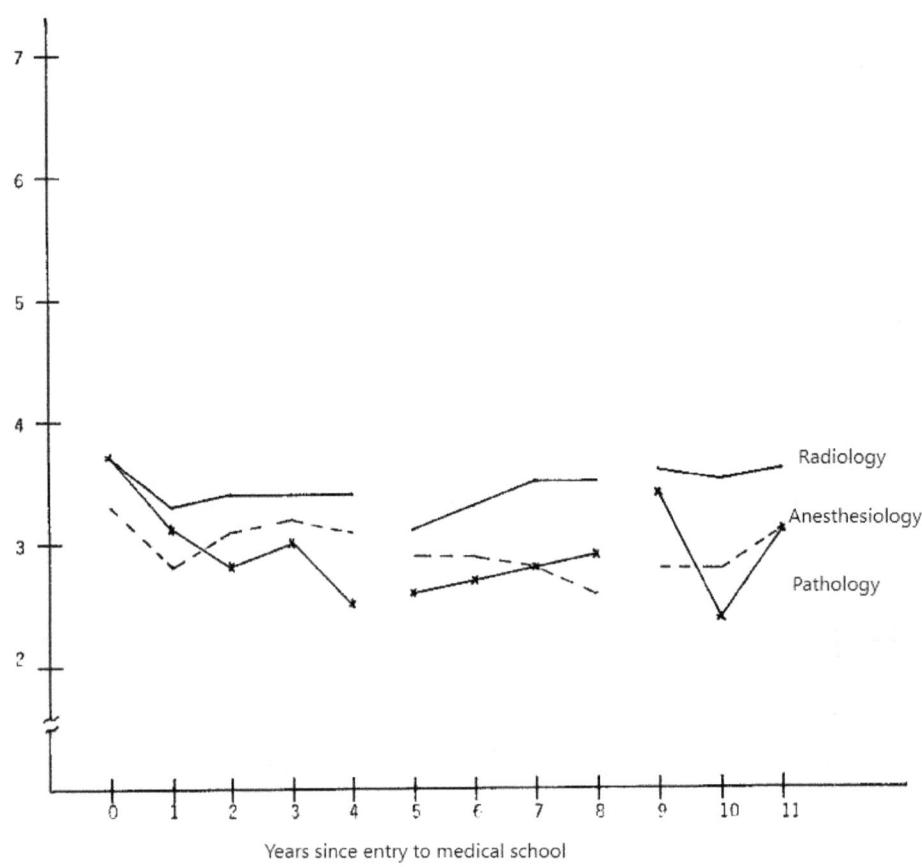

Specialty Preferences: Radiology, Anesthesiology and Pathology

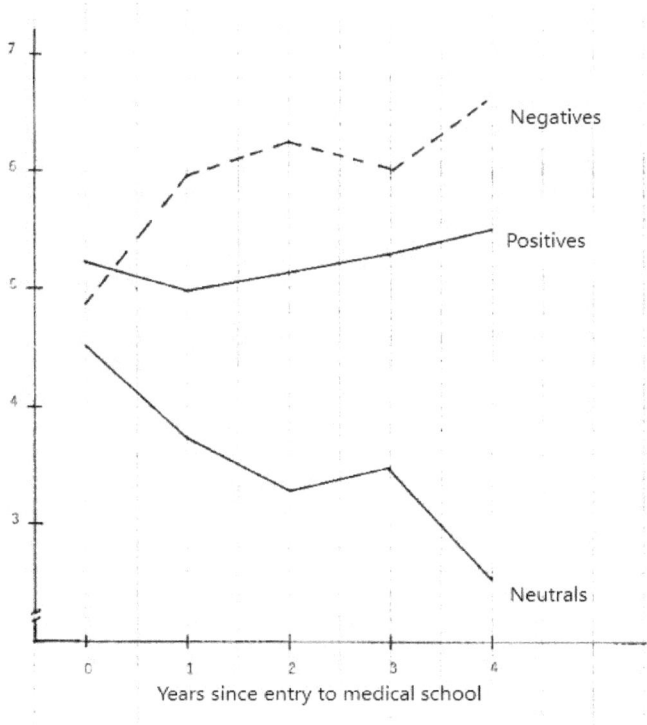

Numbers of positive, negative and neutral specialty preferences during medical school:

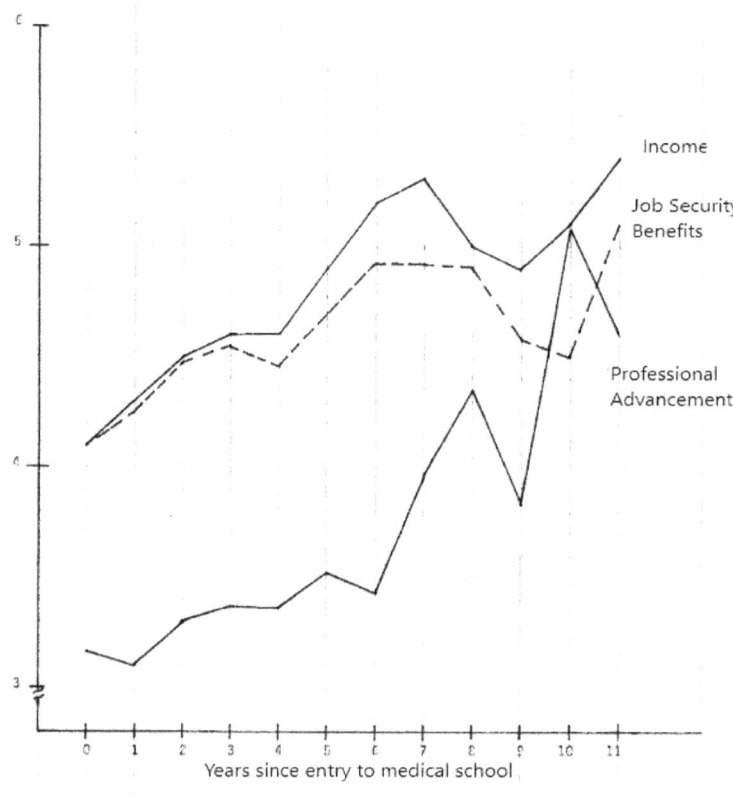

Importance of income, job security, benefits and professional advancement in decision-making.

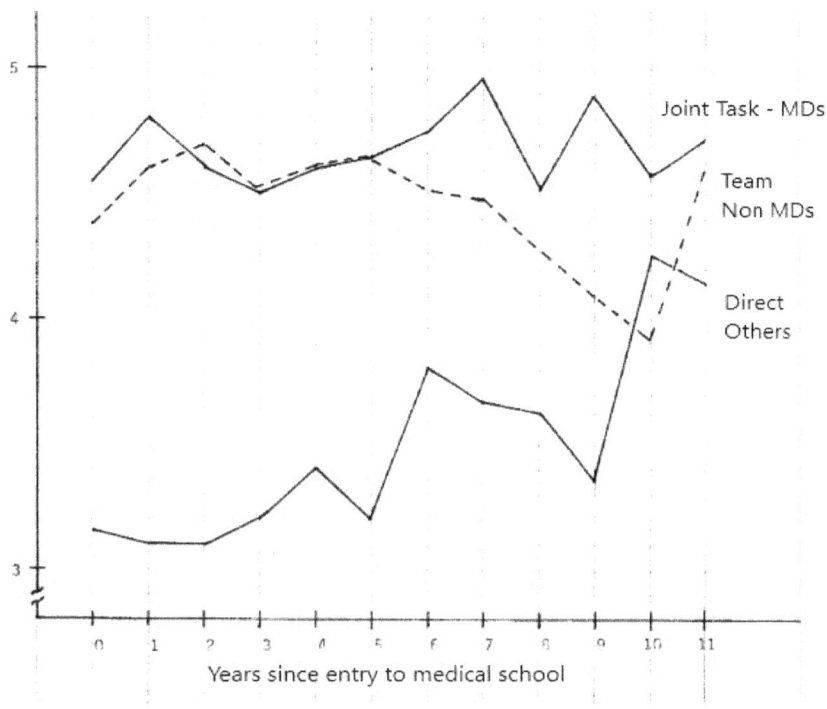

Importance of opportunities for directing others and team work with MD and Non-MD groups.

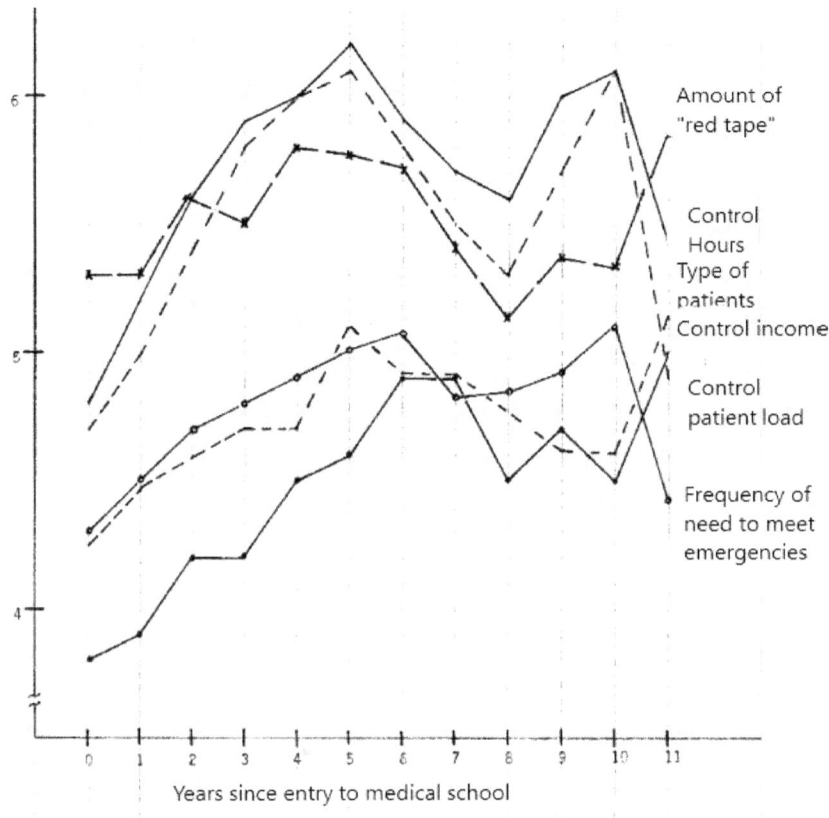

Importance of controlling patient load, hours, income, red tape, frequency of emergencies.

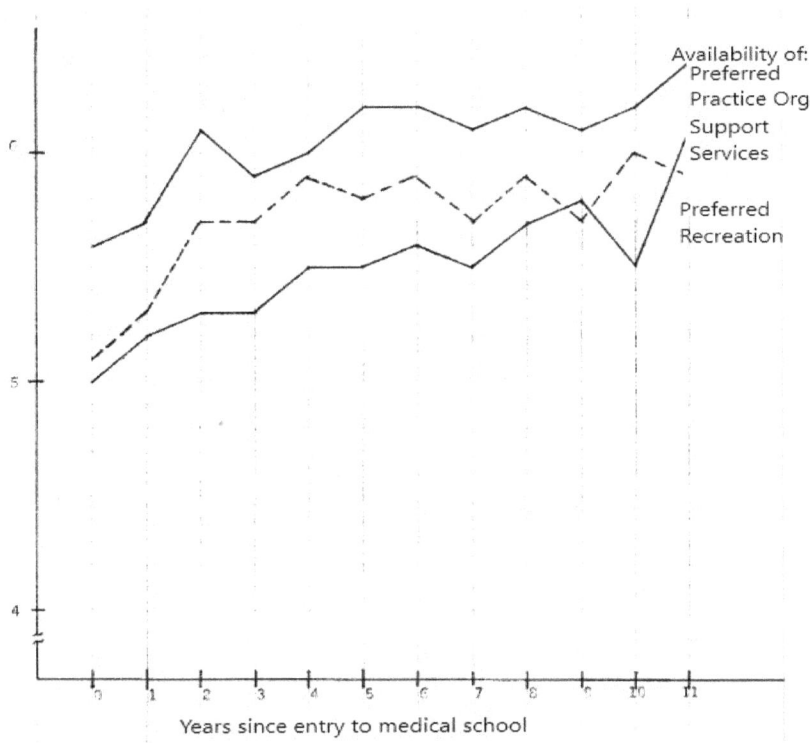

Importance of support services, desired practice organization and preferred recreation.

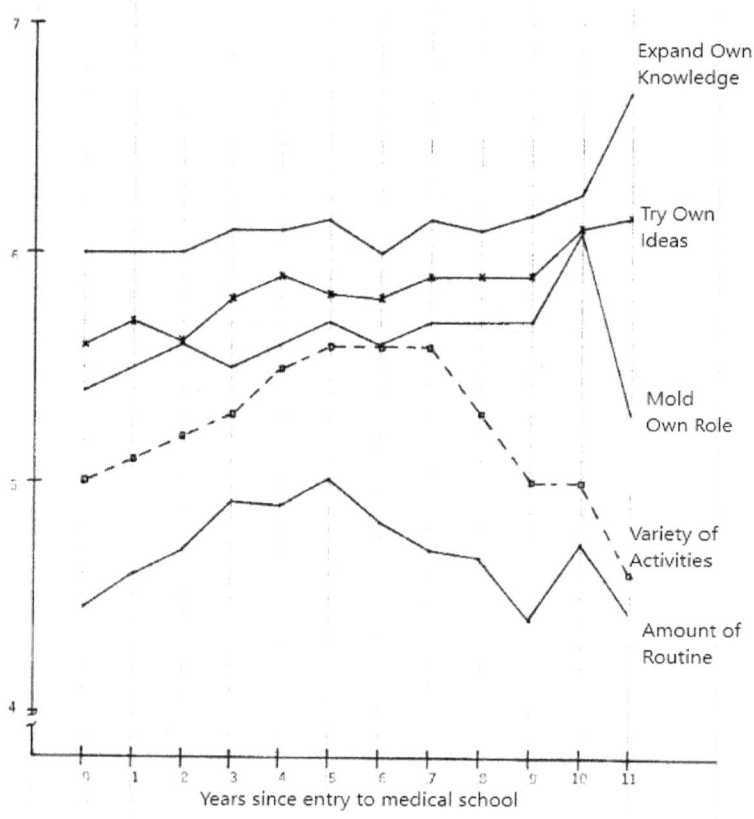

Importance of being able to expand knowledge, try ideas, mold role, etc.

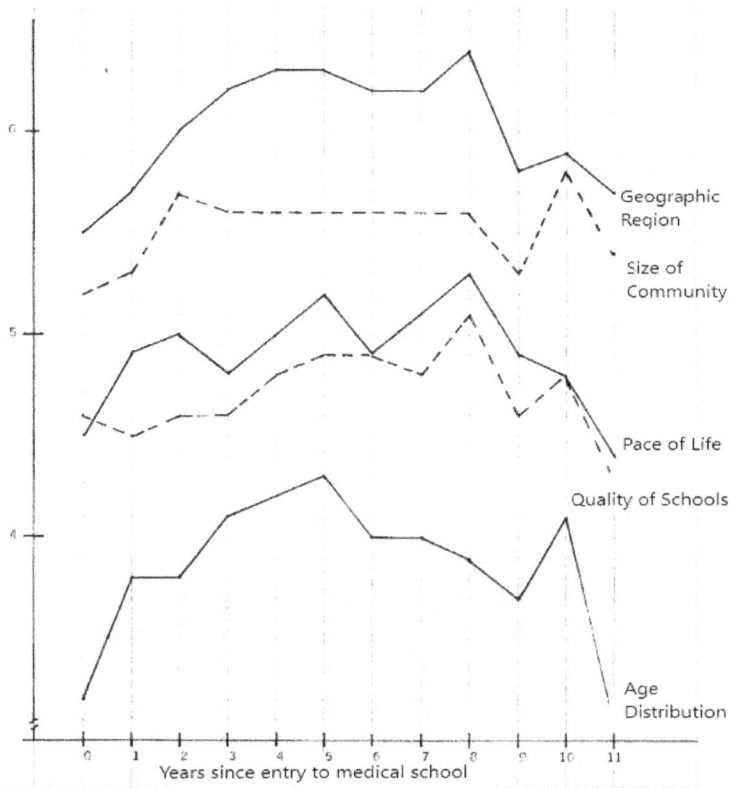

Importance of geographic region, size of community, pace of life, quality of schools and age distribution of community population in making career decisions.

Note: It should be remembered that the number of cases goes down as one gets further away from the entry time period, so the estimates of the mean are less reliable. It is probably best to mentally smooth

Biographical Questionnaire

This questionnaire was developed and modified over the years to incorporate the usual kinds of background information collected by sociologists plus some additional information that was suspected to possibly play a role in selection of medical career facets. Some of the items were included in various analyses in the course of the study but the results were mostly disappointing in that they did not show many significant association with the outcomes studied. However, with the number of categories and subcategories in many parts of the questionnaire, there would have had to have been a lot more cases in order to find any significant results. So biographical variables remain a domain for future research.

Medical School Graduates Survey

The Medical School Graduate Survey (MSG) was developed late in the course of the Longitudinal Study as we were collecting a number of graduates and decided to continue the study on into post-graduate medical education and medical practice. Unfortunately the study was terminated before we had a chance to collect and evaluate very much postgraduate data. Following medical school graduates through the course of their internships, residencies and fellowships remains an important area of research and the MSG might help future investigators in their efforts.

Physician Work-setting Instrument

The Physician Work-setting Instrument (PWSI) was developed by Naomi Quenk, PhD and Martha Albert in order to carry out a study of physicians in practice, for which a random sample of physicians in various specialties and work-settings in different communities and areas of the country was obtained from the AMA database. The intent was to develop a taxonomy of physician work-settings and relate it to career satisfaction/dissatisfaction and personality type. The questionnaire contained a set of work-setting characteristics general enough to apply to most physicians but sufficiently important as sources of satisfaction and dissatisfaction. This set of characteristics along with such features as specialty, practice organization, patient characteristics and other practice descriptors was defined as a work setting or "niche." Our intent was to administer it to our medical school graduates once they actually got into practice, but this was thwarted by the premature termination of the project.

Questionnaires

Physician Ideology Questionnaire (PIQ)

Code Number_____

Date of Administration _____

PHYSICIAN IDEOLOGY QUESTIONNAIRE

Physicians in practice today differ a great deal in what they consider to be attributes of the "ideal" physician. The purpose of this questionnaire is to sample your ideas about what the ideal physician should do and should be.

Physician Career Choice and Satisfaction

Please answer *every* item by writing in the number that corresponds to the answer that most closely represents your opinion. There are no right or wrong answers; the best answer to each question is your own personal opinion. Even if there are some items about which you feel you do not have enough knowledge to make a definite judgment, please give your best estimate based on your opinion at the present time.

Your Views About the Ideal Physician

Instructions: Please rate each of the listed statements using the scale below:

1 =Very essential 2=Usually desirable 3=Makes little or no difference

4=Usually not desirable 5=Decidedly not desirable

How Important Do You Think It Is That A Good Doctor Should:

01 __ Have control over his work setting (e. g., in a hospital or clinic)?
02 __ Have the knack of putting patients at ease?
03 __ Reserve his time in office practice for dealing with really ill persons rather than neurotic ones? 04 __ Have thorough and continually updated knowledge in the biological aspects of medicine?
05 Have the ability to deal with some of the emotional problems of patients?
06 __ Know how to utilize the services of social workers, public health nurses, and other social agency personnel in the hospital or community?
07 __ Encourage patients to express their feelings?
08 __ Have skill in applying the basic sciences of medicine to clinical practice?
09 __ Refuse to care for patients whom he feels will be uncooperative?
10 __ Supervise the allied health professionals (e. g., physical therapists, speech therapists, etc.) working with his patients?

Opinions:
This section asks for your opinions on a variety of ideas. There are no right or wrong answers. The best answer to each question is your own personal opinion.

1 =I agree very much   2=I agree a little   3= Doesn't make any difference

4=I disagree a little   5=I disagree very much

11 ___ An individual physician can contribute just as much to society by providing good clinical service as by getting involved in health-related community activities.
12 ___ Psychological factors are just as important as physical factors in the healing process.
13 ___ Most basic science research is so far removed from clinical medicine that its usefulness to the practicing physician is slight.
14 ___ Adequate treatment cannot be done unless the doctor's authority over all aspects of patient care is clearly established and preserved.
15 __ Being able to establish rapport with patients is at least as important as technical skill.
16 ___ One gets more of a feeling of accomplishment by identifying and treating a particular disease entity than by working in ill-defined or multiple problem areas.
17 __ The physician should leave the treatment of emotional, social and economic problems of patients to specialists.
18 __ A physician can effectively treat most medical problems without knowing the details of the biological processes involved.
19 __ Saying "I don't know" to a patient implies some loss of face.

20 __ The greatest contributions are made by physicians with extensive knowledge and skills in limited areas.
21 __ Of the many facets of a good physician, his knowledge of biological mechanisms is most important.
22 __ Prevention of disease as a medical activity is primarily the responsibility of health departments rather than the responsibility of the individual physician.
23 __ The paramedical professional with great skill in a particular area is more valuable to the physician than one who is relatively "undifferentiated.
24 __ Doctors have the right to expect, in return for their skilled advice and/or treatment, that patients and their families will follow orders.
25 __ A physician must imply that he knows the diagnosis in order not to destroy the patient's confidence in him.
26 __ Compassion is a luxury which the busy physician cannot afford.
27 __ Physicians who prefer to work in broad problem areas would probably not do well in more rigorous and detailed disciplines

How Important Is It For A Good Doctor To:

1=Extremely important   2=Quite important   3= Somewhat important

4=Not too important   5=Not at all important

28 __ Have the ability to deal with some of the social problems of patients?
29 __ Know how to work with non-medical specialists on a treatment team in a medical setting?
30 __ Know the effect of a patient's illness on his family?
31 __ Be adept in history taking?
32 __ Be skilled in interpersonal relations?
33 __ Have his recommendations be given precedence over those of other members of the medical or health team?
34 __ Be able and willing to talk with patients about their personal problems?
35 __ Be a leader in health planning in his community?
36 __ Make some of his time available for service to health-related community organizations?
37 __ Reassure and calm patients who are upset about their illness?
38 __ Be dignified and tactful with patients?
39 __ Know something about the private and public social and welfare agencies in his community?
40 __ Reserve his time, because of the demands of a busy practice, for the treatment of disease rather than spend time in the prevention of illness?
41 __ Adapt treatment to the special needs (emotional, social, financial, etc.) of patients?
42 __ Participate actively in organized state or city public health planning and/or public health programs?
43 __ Know how to elicit discussion of emotional reactions to illness in his patients?
44 Have skill in applying the basic ideas of psychosomatic medicine and psychiatry to the practice of clinical medicine?

Thinking About Doctors and Nurses Working In A Hospital, In General, Who Do You Think Should:

1 =Doctor much more than nurse   2=Doctor somewhat more than nurse   3= Doctor and nurse about the same
         4=Nurse somewhat more than doctor   5=Nurse much more them doctor

45 __ Be responsible for getting information about the patient's family and home situation?

46 __ Discuss post-hospital plans with the patient?
47 __ Be responsible for explaining resources for rehabilitative care to the patient?
48 __ Take the responsibility for discussing the patient's condition with his family?
49 __ Be responsible for explaining planned tests, treatment procedures, etc., to the patient?
50 __ Discuss post-hospital plans with the patient's family?

Student-Faculty Role Questionnaire Student Form (Expectations)

OTIS

STUDENT-FACULTY ROLE QUESTIONNAIRE

(Part One - Expectations)

The relationship between students and faculty differs from one college or university to another and from one department to another. The kind and quality of the relationship which is needed, valued or required at one institution may be quite different from that which is needed, valued, or required at another institution. The purpose of the Student-Faculty Role Questionnaire is to help define the nature of this relationship. You are asked, as an observer and participant in the student-faculty relations, to record your opinions and impressions of the relationships at this college. There are no right or wrong answers; the best answer to each question is your own personal opinion. If you feel that you do not really know enough about some of the items to make a definite judgment, give your best estimate based upon your experience and observations.

Please answer every item by marking in the space provided the number that corresponds to the alternative which seems to you to be most appropriate.

YOUR VIEWS ABOUT THE IDEAL STUDENT-FACULTY RELATIONSHIP

Directions: Of the things mentioned below, some are probably essential to a good relationship between students and faculty, some not desirable, and same not important at all. Attach the number representing your judgment in the space provided.

1 = very essential   2 = usually desirable   3 = makes little or no difference

4 = usually not desirable   5 = decidedly not desirable

HOW IMPORTANT IS IT TO THE IDEAL STUDENT-FACULTY RELATIONSHIP:

___ 1. That faculty members be willing to talk with students about personal matters?
___ 2. That faculty members encourage office visits for informal talks?
___ 3. That students receive recognition for their accomplishments?
___ 4. That faculty members go out of their way to be helpful to students?
___ 5. That faculty members be patient with students who do not seem to understand what is presented?

___ 6. That the individuality of students be recognized by faculty members?
___ 7. That students recognize the status of faculty members?
___ 8. That students are considerate towards faculty members?
___ 9. That students are enthusiastic about learning?
___ 10. That faculty members are friendly and supportive rather than reserved?
___ 11. That faculty members are generally cheerful and sometimes humorous?
___ 12. That an instructor pay attention to cues from students that he is not getting his information across?
___ 13. That students are meticulous and persistent in their work rather than casual and inclined to skip over details.
___ 14. That students tackle problems on their own rather than waiting for them to be brought up in class?
___ 15. That faculty members be considerate of patients they interview or examine?
___ 16. That faculty members request permission from patients for procedures to be carried out?
___ 17. That faculty members explain procedures and/or findings to patients?
___ 18. That students make suggestions or recommendations to faculty members regarding teaching materials, methods and the like?
___ 19. That faculty members try to accommodate their instructional format to student suggestions and recommendations?
___ 20. That faculty members learn about students! level of experience with the course topic prior to presentation?
___ 21. That students question facts, opinions, or interpretations of faculty members?
___ 22. That students use texts and journals to further their understanding?
___ 23. That the major part of a faculty member's interest and energy is devoted to teaching?
___ 24. That a student have free or elective time to do with what he wants?

OPINIONS

This section asks for opinions. There are no right or wrong answers; the best answer to each question is your own personal opinion.

In the space provided, mark the number 1,2,3,4, or 5, which most closely indicates your feeling about each statement.

1 = I agree very much   2 = I agree a little   3 = Doesn't make any difference

4 = I disagree a little   5 = I disagree very much

___ 25. Students who want to make their relationship with faculty members more informal, to treat them like peers, don't really understand what it means to be a student.
___ 26. Students should **not** be allowed to participate in the planning of any educational sessions since they lack the experience and would probably not get the material across effectively. Besides, it would be a very inefficient use of time.
___ 27. When he is introduced to a patient, a medical student should be clearly identified as a student.

HOW IMPORTANT IS IT TO YOU THAT YOU BE ABLE TO DO EACH OF THE FOLLOWING:

1 = Extremely important   2 = Quite important   3 = Somewhat important

4 = Not at all important   5 = Not at all important

___ 28. Be punctual?
___ 29. Show interest in your course material?
___ 30. Seek out faculty members for informal discussions?

___ 31. Include faculty members in social and unofficial academic affairs?
___ 32. Show your appreciation to faculty members who make an effort to do well by you?
___ 33. Respect faculty members who are trying to increase your understanding of the complexities of the world?
___ 34. Really invest yourself in the work of a course?
___ 35. Give serious consideration to what faculty members say?

HOW IMPORTANT IS IT TO YOU THAT FACULTY MEMBERS:

1 = Very essential 2 = Usually desirable 3 = Makes little or no difference

4 = Usually not desirable 5 = Decidedly not desirable

___ 36. Understand and appreciate you as an individual?
___ 37. Talk with you on a one-to-one basis?
___ 38. Help you to understand yourself?
___ 39. Help you work out problems (personal or academic)?
___ 40. Excite your curiosity through teaching?
___ 41. Let you know what is required to meet their expectations?
___ 42. Respect your individual interests in learning!
___ 43. Accommodate to student needs in teaching sessions!
___ 44. Encourage student questions and discussion?
___ 45. Give prompt feedback to students regarding their performance?
___ 46. Have their courses well organized?
___ 47. Be good examples in their dealings with patients?
___ 48. Evaluate you on a continuous grading system (A,B,C,D,F) as opposed to a pass-fail system?
___ 49. Are good speakers or lecturers?
___ 50. Provide a syllabus or outline at the beginning of a course or block?

HOW IMPORTANT IS IT TO YOU:

1 = Extremely important 2 = Quite important 3 = Somewhat important

4 = Not too important 5 = Not at all important

___ 51 To understand and use the concepts which are presented to you?
___ 52. For classes or laboratories to be orderly and productive at all times?
___ 53. To provide a service when you are assigned to a ward or clinic?
___ 54. To do some of the teaching?
___ 55. To be taught about "emergency medicine" (i. e., medical care during disasters and wartime)?
___ 56. To become a good clinician rather than a good researcher?
___ 57. To become a good teacher rather than to become a good clinician?
___ 58. To be theoretically oriented rather than practically oriented?
___ 59. To specialize rather than go into general medicine?
___ 60. To learn how to elicit information from patients.
___ 61. To be taught how to work with non-medical specialists in caring for patients?
___ 62. To take advantage of summer work positions to develop research skills and knowledge rather than to get experience working with patients?
___ 63. To learn about medical care outside of the usual medical setting (e. g. in the community)?
___ 64. That faculty members get to know you fairly well?

HOW IMPORTANT SHOULD IT BE, AT THIS SCHOOL, FOR STUDENTS:

1 = Extremely important   2 = Quite important   3 = Somewhat important

4 = Not too important   5 = Not at all important

___ 65. To learn to better understand themselves?
___ 66. To find purpose or meaning in their professional roles?
___ 67. To learn to understand the complexities of the world?
___ 68. To learn to appreciate the beauty in life?
___ 69. To show academic scholarship?
___ 70. To endeavor to master the basic sciences?
___ 71. To be interested in the social context of medical care?
___ 72. To become able to function in any general area of medicine?
___ 73. To learn how to educate themselves?
___ 74. To develop a psychological awareness of patients?
___ 75. To learn how to prepare patients, emotionally, for examinations or the use of instruments?
___ 76. To appreciate the sociocultural aspects of health and disease?
___ 77. To learn how to communicate findings to patients?
___ 78. To develop clinical judgment or intuition?

HOW IMPORTANT IS IT TO THE IDEAL STUDENT - FACULTY RELATIONSHIP:

1 = Very essential   2 = Usually desirable   3 = Makes little or no difference

4 = Usually not desirable   5 = Decidedly not desirable

___ 79. That students be informed about revisions in school policy?
___ 80. That students be informed regarding issues of conflict within the school?

HOW IMPORTANT IS IT TO YOUR RELATIONSHIP WITH FACULTY MEMBERS:

1 = Extremely important   2 = Quite important   3 = Somewhat important

4 = Not too important   5 = Not at all important

___ 81. That they have a good reputation in their field!
___ 82. That they be involved in research personally?
___ 83. That they be involved in clinical practice personally?
___ 84. That they participate in community affairs?
___ 85. That they participate in medical school affairs (outside of their own department)!

IN GENERAL, WHO DO YOU THINK SHOULD HAVE MORE INFLUENCE:

Physician Career Choice and Satisfaction

1 = Faculty member much more than student
2 = Faculty member somewhat more
3 = Faculty member and student about the same
4 = Student somewhat more than faculty member
5 = Student much more than faculty member

___ 86. In determining educational methods?
___ 87. In determining educational objectives?
___ 88. In preparing educational materials?
___ 89. In choosing professional goals!
___ 90. In relations with administrative personnel?
___ 91. In specifying methods of study or learning?
___ 92. In providing instruction?
___ 93. In deciding what is important to learn?

Student-Faculty Role Questionnaire Student Form (Perceptions)

OTIS

STUDENT-FACULTY ROLE QUESTIONNAIRES

(Part Two - Perceptions)

YOUR VIEWS ABOUT STUDENT-FACULTY RELATIONSHIPS **AT THIS SCHOOL**

This section asks you to give your impressions of various aspects of the student- faculty relationship at this school. Please make a judgment on every item even though you may feel your ratings are based on limited exposure to the groups in question . We are interested in your impressions based on the experience you have had up to this point.

WHAT PROPORTION OF THE FACULTY WITH WHOM YOU HAVE DEALT AT THIS SCHQOL:

1 = Almost all   2 = Over half   3 = About half

4 = Less than half   5 = Very few

___ 94. Are willing to talk with students about personal matters?
___ 95. Encourage students to visit their office for informal talks?
___ 96. Give students recognition when they accomplish something?
___ 97. Go out of their way to be helpful to students?
___ 98. Are patient with students who don't seem to understand what is presented?
___ 99. Recognize the individuality of students?
___ 100. Are friendly and supportive rather than reserved?
___ 101. Are generally cheerful and sometimes humorous?
___ 102. Are considerate of patients they interview or examine?
___ 103. Request permission from patients for procedures to be carried out?
___ 104. Explain procedures and/or findings to patients?

___ 105. Try to accommodate their instructional format to student suggestions and recommendations?
___ 106. Learn about students' level of experience with the course topic prior to presentation?
___ 107. Devote the major part of their interest and energy to teaching?
___ 108. Pay attention to cues from students that they are not getting their material across?

WHAT PROPORTION OF THE STUDENTS YOU KNOW AT THIS SCHOOL:

1 = Almost all   2 = Over half   3 = About half

4 = Less than half   5 = Very few

___ 109. Pay little or no attention to the status of faculty members?
___ 110. Are considerate towards faculty members?
___ 112. Are enthusiastic about learning?
___ 113. Are meticulous and persistent in their work rather than casual and inclined to skip over details?
___ 114. Tackle problems on their own rather than wait for them to be brought up in class?
___ 115. Make suggestions or recommendations to faculty members regarding teaching materials, methods and the like?
___ 116. Question facts, opinions, or interpretations of faculty members?
___ 117. Use texts and journals to further their understanding?
___ 118. Are late for appointments, classes, etc.?
___ 119. Seek out faculty members for informal discussions?
___ 120. Show interest in course material?
___ 121. Include faculty members in social or unofficial academic affairs?
___ 122. Show their appreciation to faculty members who make an effort to do well by them?
___ 123. Respect faculty members who try to increase their understanding of the complexities of the world?
___ 124. Really invest themselves in the work bf a course?
___ 125. Seriously consider what faculty members say?

WHAT PROPORTION OF THE FACULTY WITH WHOM YOU HAVE DEALT AT THIS SCHOOL:

1 = Almost all   2 = Over half   3 = About half

4 = Less than half   5 = Very few

___ 126. Know you fairly well?
___ 127. Understand and appreciate students as individuals?
___ 128. Talk with students on a one-to-one basis?
___ 129. Help students understand themselves?
___ 130. Help students work out personal or academic problems?
___ 131. Excite the curiosity of students through their teaching?
___ 132. Let students know what is required to meet their expectations?
___ 133. Respect individual interests in learning?
___ 134. Accommodate to student needs in teaching sessions?
___ 135. Set aside free or elective time for students to do with what they want?
___ 136. Encourage student questions and discussion?
___ 137. Give prompt feedback to students regarding their performance?
___ 138. Have their courses well organized?
___ 139. Evaluate students on a continuous grading system (A,B,C,D,F) as opposed to a pass-fail system?

___ 140. Are good speakers or lecturers?

WHAT PROPORTION OF THE STUDENTS YOU KNOW AT THIS SCHOOL:

1 = Almost all   2 = Over half   3 = About half

4 = Less than half   5 = Very few

___ 141. Understand and use the concepts which are presented to them?
___ 142. Have provided a service when assigned to a ward or clinic?
___ 143. Take advantage of summer work positions to develop research skills?
___ 144. Take advantage of summer work positions to get experience working with patients?

HOW MUCH EMPHASIS DOES THIS SCHOOL, AS A WHOLE, PLACE ON STUDENTS:

1 = Major emphasis   2 = Substantial emphasis   3 = Some emphasis

4 = Hardly any emphasis   5 = No emphasis

___ 145. Learning to better understand themselves?
___ 146. Finding purpose or meaning in their professional roles?
___ 147. Learning to understand the complexities of the world?
___ 148. Learning to appreciate the beauty in life?
___ 149. Showing academic scholarship?
___ 150. Mastering the basic sciences?
___ 151. Being interested in the social context of medical care?
___ 152. Being able to function in any general area of medicine?
___ 153. Learning how to educate themselves?
___ 154. Developing a psychological awareness of patients?
___ 155. Learning how to prepare patients, emotionally, for examinations or the use of instruments?
___ 156. Appreciating the sociocultural aspects of health and disease?
___ 157. Learning how to communicate findings to patients?
___ 158. Developing clinical judgment or intuition?
___ 159. Learning how to elicit information from patients?
___ 160. Learning how to work with non-medical specialists in caring for patients?

WHAT PROPORTION OF THE FACULTY WITH WHOM YOU HAVE DEALT AT THIS SCHOOL.:

1 = Almost all   2 = Over half   3 = About half

4 = Less than half   5 = Very few

___ 161. Provide a syllabus or outline at the beginning of a course or block?
___ 162. Have orderly and productive teaching sessions (classes, laboratories, supervisory sessions, etc.)?
___ 163. Have a good reputation in their field?
___ 164. Are involved in research?
___ 165. Are involved in clinical practice?
___ 166. Participate in community affairs?

___ 167. Participate in medical school affairs (outside of their own department)?
___ 168. Inform students about revisions in school policy?
___ 169. Inform students regarding issues of conflict within the school?
___ 170. Allow students to do some of the teaching?
___ 171. Emphasize theoretical rather than practical matters?

HOW MUCH EMPHASIS DOES THIS SCHOOL, AS A WHOLE, PLACE ON:

1 = Major emphasis   2 = Substantial emphasis   3 = Some emphasis

4 = Hardly any emphasis   5 = No emphasis

___ 172. "Emergency medicine" (i. e., medical care during disasters and wartime)?
___ 173. Clinical work?
___ 174. Research work?
___ 175. Specialization?
___ 176. Medical care outside of the usual medical settings?

IN GENERAL WHO HAS THE MORE INFLUENCE IN THIS SCHOOL.:

1 = Faculty much more than students   2 = Faculty somewhat more

3 = Faculty and students about the same   4 = Students somewhat more

5 = Students much more than faculty

___ 177. In determining educational methods?
___ 178. In determining educational objectives?
___ 179. In preparing educational materials?
___ 180. In choosing professional goals?
___ 181. In relations with administrative personnel?
___ 182. In specifying methods of study or learning?
___ 183. In providing instruction?
___ 184. In deciding what is important to learn?

Student-Faculty Role Questionnaire Faculty Form (Expectations)

OTIS

STUDENT-FACULTY ROLE QUESTIONNAIRE

(Part 1 - Expectations)

The relationship between students and faculty differs from one college or university to another and from one department to another. The kind and quality of the relationship which is needed, valued, or required at one institution may be quite different from that which is needed, valued, or required at another institution, The purpose of the Student-Faculty Role Questionnaire is to help define the nature of this relationship, You are asked, as an observer and participant in student-faculty relations to record your opinions and impressions of the relationships at this college, There are no right or wrong answers; the best answer to each question is your own personal opinion, If you feel that you do not really know enough about some of the items to make a definite judgment, give your best estimate based upon your experience and observations.

Please answer every item by marking in the space provided the number that corresponds to the alternative that seems to you to be most appropriate,

YOUR VIEWS ABOUT THE IDEAL STUDENT-FACULTY RELATIONSHIP

Directions: Of the things mentioned below, some are probably essential to a good relationship between students and faculty, some not desirable, and some not important at all. In the space provided, mark the number 1,2,3,4, or 5, to indicate your opinion of the thing mentioned.

1 = very essential   2 = usually desirable   3 = makes little or no difference

4 = usually not desirable   5 = decidedly not desirable

HOW IMPORTANT IS IT TO THE IDEAL STUDENT-FACULTY RELATIONSHIP:

__ 1. That faculty members be willing to talk with students about personal matters?
__ 2. That faculty members encourage office visits for informal talks?
__ 3. That students receive recognition for their accomplishments?
__ 4. That faculty members go out of their way to be helpful to students?
__ 5. That faculty members be patient with students who do not seem to under- stand what is presented?
__ 6. That the individuality of students be recognized by faculty members?
__ 7. That students recognize the status of faculty members?
__ 8. That students are considerate toward faculty members?
__ 9. That students are enthusiastic about learning?
__ 10. That faculty members are friendly and supportive rather than reserved?
__ 11. That faculty members are generally cheerful and sometimes humorous?
__ 12. That faculty members appear polished and sophisticated in their dealings with others (students, patients, other faculty)?
__ 13. That students appear confident, adventurous, "thick-skinned", rather than shy, mild-mannered or timid?
__ 14. That students are meticulous and persistent in their work rather than casual and inclined to skip over details?
__ 15. That students tackle problems on their own rather than waiting for them to be brought up in class?
__ 16. That faculty members be considerate of patients they interview or examine?
__ 17. That faculty members request permission from patients for procedures to be carried out?
__ 18. That faculty members explain procedures and/or findings to patients?
__ 19. That students make suggestions or recommendations to faculty members regarding teaching materials, methods and the like?
__ 20. That faculty members try to accommodate their instructional format to student suggestions and recommendations?
__ 21. That faculty members learn about students' level of experience with the course topic prior to presentation?
__ 22. That students question facts, opinions, or interpretations of faculty members?
__ 23. That students use texts and journals to further their understanding?
__ 24. That the major part of a faculty member's interest and energy is devoted to teaching?

___ 25. That a faculty member have a thorough knowledge of his subject matter?
___ 26. That a student have free or elective time to do with what he wants?

OPINIONS

This section asks for opinions. There are no right or wrong answers; the best answer to each question is your own personal opinion.

In the space provided, mark the number 1, 2, 3, 4, or 5, which most closely indicates your feeling about each statement.

1 = I agree very much   2 = I agree a little   3 = Doesn't make any difference

4 = I disagree a little   5 = I disagree very much

___ 27. Faculty members should work with students, rather than above them,
___ 28. Faculty members who want to make their relationship with students more informal, to treat them as peers, don't really understand what it means to be a teacher.
___ 29. In general, a faculty member is better off being cautious and prudent when dealing with student demands or pleas rather than being trusting and sympathetic.
___ 30. Students should not be allowed to participate in the planning of any educational sessions since they lack experience and would probably not get the material across effectively. Besides, it would be a very inefficient use of the time.
___ 31. If students want to know about points of view different from that held by a faculty member, they should find out on their own.

HOW IMPORTANT TO YOU IS IT THAT STUDENTS:

1 = Extremely important   2 = Quite important   3 = Somewhat important

4 = Not too important   5 = Not at all important

___ 32. Be punctual?
___ 33. Show interest in : our course material?
___ 34. Seek you out for informal discussions?
___ 35. Include you in social and unofficial academic affairs?
___ 36. Invite you to their homes?
___ 37. Appreciate your efforts to do well by them?
___ 38. Care whether or not you are trying to increase their understanding of the complexities of the world?
___ 39. Really invest themselves in the work of your course?
___ 40. Give serious consideration to what you sa1y?

HOW IMPORTANT IS IT TO YOU THAT YOU BE ABLE TO DO EACH OF THE FOLLOWING:

1 = Very essential   2 = Usually desirable   3 = Makes little or no difference

4 = Usually not desirable   5 = Decidedly not desirable

___ 41. Understand and appreciate students as individuals?
___ 42. Talk with students on a one-to-one basis?

___ 43. Help students to understand themselves?
___ 44. Help students to work out their problems (personal or academic)?
___ 45. Invite students to your home?
___ 46. Excite the curiosity of students through teaching?
___ 47. Let students know what is required to meet your expectations of them?
___ 48. Take account of individual interests in learning when you plan a course?
___ 49. Accommodate to student needs in teaching sessions?
___ 50. Elicit student questions and discussion?
___ 51. Give prompt feedback to students regarding their performance?
___ 52. Have your teaching materials and format well organized?
___ 53. Evaluate students by means of regular tests as opposed to only at the end of a section?
___ 54. Evaluate students on a continuous grading system (A,B,C,D,F) as opposed to a pass-fail system?
___ 55. Evaluate all of a students performances?
___ 56. Evaluate students only on the basis of objective standards?
___ 57. Be a good speaker or lecturer?

HOW IMPORTANT IS IT TO YOU THAT STUDENTS:

1 = Extremely important   2 = Quite important   3 = Somewhat important

4 = Not too important   5 = Not at all important

___ 58. Understand and use concepts which are presented to them?
___ 59. Are orderly and productive at all times in classes or laboratories?
___ 60. Take care of some of the menial tasks when they are assigned to a service?
___ 61. Provide a service function when assigned to a ward or clinic?
___ 62. Do some of the teaching?
___ 63. Be taught about "emergency medicine" (i,e,, medical care during disasters and wartime)?
___ 64. Become good clinicians rather than good researchers?
___ 65. Become good teachers rather than good clinicians?
___ 66. Pay attention to the practical management of problems?
___ 67. Concentrate most of their time on evaluation and treatment of specific disease processes?
___ 68. Be trained for specialties rather than general medicine?
___ 69. Be taught how to elicit information from patients?
___ 70. Learn how to use information from non-medical specialists?
___ 71. Learn how to make use of the various community agencies in their treatment of patients?
___ 72. Be more interested in theory than practical application?

HOW IMPORTANT SHOULD IT BE, AT THIS SCHOOL, FOR STUDENTS:

1 = Extremely important   2 = quite important   3 = Somewhat important

4 = Not too important   5 = Not at all important

___ 73. To learn to better understand themselves?
___ 74. To find purpose or meaning in their professional roles?
___ 75. To learn to understand the complexities of the world?
___ 76. To learn to appreciate the beauty in life?
___ 77. To show academic scholarship?

___ 78. To endeavor to master the basic sciences?
___ 79. To be interested in the social context of medical care?
___ 80. To become able to function in any general area of medicine?
___ 81. To learn how to educate themselves?
___ 82. To know specific facts rather than general principles?
___ 83. To develop a psychological awareness of patients?
___ 84. To learn how to prepare patients, emotionally, for examinations and the use of instruments?
___ 85. To appreciate the sociocultural aspects of health and disease?
___ 86. To learn how to communicate findings to patients?
___ 87. To develop clinical judgment or intuition?

HOW IMPORTANT IS IT TO THE IDEAL STUDENT-FACULTY RELATIONSHIP:

1 = Very essential   2 = Usually desirable   3 = Makes little or no difference

4 = Usually not desirable   5 = Decidedly not desirable

___ 88. That students do not hinder house staff in performing their duties?
___ 89. That students be informed about revisions in school policy?
___ 90. That students be informed regarding issues of conflict within the school?
___ 91. That faculty members locate opportunities for students to get summer work experience in the profession?

HOW IMPORTANT IS IT TO YOUR RELATIONSHIP WITH STUDENTS:

1 = Extremely important   2 = Quite important   3 = Somewhat important

4 = Not too important   5 = Not at all important

___ 92. That you "get ahead" professionally?
___ 93. That you be involved in research personally'?
___ 94. That you be involved in clinical practice personally?
___ 95. That you participate in community affairs?
___ 96. That you participate in medical school affairs (outside of your own department)?
___ 97. That they (students) be involved in extracurricular affairs?
___ 98. That they (students) be free of demands outside of school?

IN GENERAL. WHO DO YOU THINK SHOULD HAVE MORE INFLUENCE:

1 = Faculty member much more than student   2 = Faculty member somewhat more

3 = Faculty member and student about the same   4 = Student somewhat more than faculty member

5 = Student much more than faculty member

___ 99. In determining educational methods?
___ 100. In determining educational objectives?
___ 101. In preparing educational materials?
___ 102. In choosing professional goals?
___ 103. In relations with administrative personnel?
___ 104. In specifying methods of study or learning?

__ 105. In promoting good relations between students and faculty?
__ 106. In providing instruction?
__ 107. In deciding what is important to learn?

Student-Faculty Role Questionnaire Faculty Form (Perceptions)

OTIS

STUDENT-FACULTY ROLE QUESTIONNAIRE

(Part Two - Perceptions))

YOUR VIEWS ABOUT STUDENT-FACULTY RELATIONSHIPS **AT THIS SCHOOL**

This section asks you to give your impressions of various aspects of the student-faculty relationship at this school, Please make a judgment on every item even though you may feel your ratings are based on limited exposure to the groups in question, We are interested in your impressions based on the experience you have had up to this point.

WHAT PROPORTION OF THE FACULTY YOU KNOW AT THIS SCHOOL:

1 = Almost all   2 = Over half   3 = About half

4 = Less than half   5 = Very few

__ 108. Are willing to talk with students about personal matters?
__ 109. Encourage students to visit their office for informal talks?
__ 110. Give students recognition when they accomplish something?
__ 111. Go out of their way to be helpful to students?
__ 112. Are patient with students who don't seem to understand what is presented?
__ 113. Recognize the individuality of students?
__ 114. Are friendly and supportive rather than reserved?
__ 115. Are generally cheerful and sometimes humorous?
__ 116. Appear polished and sophisticated in their dealings with others?
__ 117. Are considerate of patients they interview or examine?
__ 118. Request permission from patients for procedures to be carried out?
__ 119. Explain procedures and/or findings to patients?
__ 120. Try to accommodate their instructional format to student suggestions and recommendations?
__ 121. Learn about students' level of experience with the course topic prior to presentation?
__ 122. Devote the major part of their interest and energy to teaching?
__ 123. Have a thorough knowledge of their subject matter?

WHAT PROPORTION OF THE STUDENTS WITH WHOM YOU HAVE DEALT AT THIS SCHOOL:

l = Almost all   2 = Over half   3 = About half

4 = Less than half   5 = Very few

___ 124. Pay little or no attention to the status of faculty members?
___ 125. Are considerate towards faculty members?
___ 126. Are enthusiastic about learning?
___ 127. Present themselves as confident, adventurous, "thick-skinned," rather than shy, mild-mannered or timid?
___ 128. Are meticulous and persistent in their work rather than casual and inclined to skip over details?

WHAT PROPORTION OF THE STUDENTS WITH WHOM YOU HAVE DEALT AT THIS SCHOOL:

1 = Almost all   2 = Over half   3 = About half

4 = Less than half   5 = Very few

___ 129. Tackle problems on their own rather than wait for them to be brought up in class?
___ 130. Make suggestions or recommendations to faculty members regarding teaching materials, methods and the like?
___ 131. Question facts, opinions, or interpretations of faculty members?
___ 132. Use texts and journals to further their understanding?
___ 133. Are late for appointments, classes, etc,?
___ 134. Seek out faculty members for informal discussions?
___ 135. Show interest in course material?
___ 136. Include faculty members in social or unofficial academic affairs?
___ 137. Show their appreciation to faculty members who make an effort to do well by them?
___ 138. Respect faculty members who try to increase their understanding of the complexities of the world?
___ 139. Really invest themselves in the work of a course?
___ 140. Seriously consider what faculty members say?

WHAT PROPORTION OF THE FACULTY YOU KNOW: AT THIS SCHOOL:

1 = Almost all   2 = Over half   3 = About half

4 = Less than half   5 = Very few

___ 141. Understand and appreciate students as individuals?
___ 142. Talk with students on a one-to-one basis?
___ 143. Help students understand themselves?
___ 144. Help students work out personal or academic problems?
___ 145. Invite students to their homes?
___ 146. Excite the curiosity of students through their teaching?
___ 147. Let students know what is required to meet their expectations?
___ 148. Respect individual interests in learning?
___ 149. Accommodate to student needs in teaching sessions?
___ 150. Set aside free or elective time for students to do with what they want?
___ 151. Encourage student questions and discussion?
___ 152. Give prompt feedback to students regarding their performance?
___ 153. Have their courses well organized?
___ 154. Evaluate students by means of regular tests as opposed to only at the end of a section?
___ 155. Evaluate students on a continuous grading system (A,B,C,D,F) as opposed to a pass-fail system?
___ 156. Evaluate all of a student's performances, even if there are several instructors?

___ 157. Evaluate students only on the basis of objective standards?
___ 158. Are good speakers or lecturers?

WHAT PROPORTION OF THE STUDENTS WITH WHOM YOU HAVE DEALT AT THIS SCHOOL:

1 = Almost all   2 = Over half   3 = About half

4 = Less than half   5 = Very few

___ 159. Understand and use the concepts which are presented to them?
___ 160. Have avoided doing menial tasks when assigned to a service?

WHAT PROPORTION OF THE STUDENTS WITH WHOM YOU HAVE DEALT AT THIS SCHOOL:

1 = Almost all   2 = Over half   2 = About half

4 = Less than half   5 = Very few

___ 161. Have provided a service when assigned to a ward or clinic?
___ 162. Interfere with house staff in the performance of their duties?
___ 163. Are free of demands outside of school?
___ 164. Are involved in extracurricular affairs?
___ 165. Invite faculty members to their homes?
___ 166. Take advantage of summer work positions to develop research skills?
___ 167. Take advantage of summer work positions to get experience working with patients?

HOW MUCH EMPHASIS DOES THIS SCHOOL, **AS A WHOLE**, PLACE ON STUDENTS:

1 = Major emphasis   2 = Substantial emphasis   3 = Some emphasis

4 = Hardly any emphasis   5 = No emphasis

___ 168. Learning to better understand themselves?
___ 169. Finding purpose or meaning in their professional roles?
___ 170. Learning to understand the complexities of the world?
___ 171. Learning to appreciate the beauty in life?
___ 172. Showing academic scholarship?
___ 173. Mastering the basic sciences?
___ 174. Being interested in the social context of medical care?
___ 175. Being able to function in any general area of medicine?
___ 176. Learning how to educate themselves?
___ 177. Knowing specific facts rather than general principles?
___ 178. Developing a psychological awareness of patients?
___ 179. Learning how to prepare patients, emotionally, for examinations or the use of instruments?
___ 180. Appreciating the sociocultural aspects of health and disease?
___ 181. Learning how to communicate findings to patients?
___ 182. Developing clinical judgment or intuition?
___ 183. Learning how to elicit information from patients?

___ 184. Learning how to work with non-medical specialists in caring for patients?

WHAT PROPORTION OF THE FACULTY YOU KNOW AT THIS SCHOOL:

1 = Almost all   2 = Over half   3 = About half

4 = Less than half   5 = Very few

___ 185. Have orderly and productive teaching sessions (classes, laboratories, supervisory sessions, etc.)?
___ 186. Locate opportunities for students to get summer work experience in the profession?
___ 187. Have a good reputation in their field?
___ 188. Are involved in research?
___ 189. Are involved in clinical practice?
___ 190. Participate in community affairs?
___ 191. Participate in medical school affairs (outside of their own department)?

WHAT PROPORTION OF THE FACULTY YOU KNOW AT THIS SCHOOL:

1 = Almost all   2 = Over half   3 = About half

4 = Less than half   5 = Very few

___ 192. Inform students about revisions in school policy?
___ 193. Inform students regarding issues of conflict within the school?
___ 194. Allow students to do some of the teaching?
___ 195. Emphasize theoretical rather than practical matters?

HOW MUCH EMPHASIS DOES THIS SCHOOL, **AS A WHOLE**, PLACE ON:

1 = Major emphasis   2 = Substantial emphasis   3 = Some emphasis

4 = Hardly any emphasis   5 = No emphasis

___ 196. "Emergency medicine" (i. e., medical care during disasters and wartime)?
___ 197. Clinical work?
___ 198. Research work?
___ 199. Specialization?
___ 200. Medical care outside of the usual medical settings?

IN GENERAL WHO HAS THE MORE INFLUENCE IN THIS SCHOOL:

1 = Faculty much more than students   2 = Faculty somewhat more

3 = Faculty and students about the same   4 = Students somewhat more

5 = Students much more than faculty

___ 201. In determining educational methods?
___ 202. In determining educational objectives?

Physician Career Choice and Satisfaction

__ 203. In preparing educational materials?
__ 204. In choosing professional goals?
__ 205. In relations with administrative personnel?
__ 206. In specifying methods of study or learning?
__ 207. In promoting good relations between students and faculty?
__ 208. In providing instruction?
__ 209. In deciding what is important to learn?

Clerkship Socialization Intensity Questionnaire

CLERKSHIP QUESTIONNAIRE

For questions 1 through 9 below, please rate each of your required and elective/selective clerkships using the following scale:

1 = Not at all   2 = To a very small extent   3 = To some extent   4 = To a moderate extent

5 = To a large extent   6 = To a great extent   7 = To a very great extent

(Please write in the name of your electives and selectives)

On your rotation, to what extent:	Med	Ob-Gyn	Ped	Psy	Surg			
1. were you permitted to make decisions and take responsibility for patients?								
2. was there agreement among your supervisors about appropriate treatments and procedures?								
3. was it common for someone to observe you doing some task and make comments about your performance or how you could have performed it?								
4. did you feel your duties were central to the practice of the specialty?								
5. did you have direct contact with faculty supervisors?								
6. did you have informal contact (off the service) with supervisors?								

7. did you have control over or a choice about your training experience?									
8. did faculty have a definite idea of what they wanted you to learn?									
9. was your feedback concerned with your general abilities as a physician?									
10. was your feedback concerned with your skills in the particular specialty?									
11. was your feedback concerned with irrelevant matters?									

12. On which rotations, if any, did you have an experience that really "turned you on" (+) or really turned you off (-) to that particular area of medicine? (Please list those rotations with a + or – to indicate the quality of experience)

_____
—
_____
—
_____
—
_____
—

13. Did you have a clerkship, preceptorship, selective or elective in any of the following settings? (Please check those that apply)

____ Physician's office (solo practice)
____ Small group practice
____ Large group practice (e. g., Lovelace)
____ Urban outpatient health clinic (e. g., Family Health Center)
____ Rural outpatient health clinic (e. g., Porvenir)
____ Private hospital
____ City/county/state hospital (other than BCMC)
____ VA hospital
____ Military hospital
____ Public Health Service
____ Student Health Service

14. During medical school, did you have any significant amount of exposure to any of the following types of physician? (Please check those that apply)

Physician Career Choice and Satisfaction

___ Family Physician
___ Allergist
___ Anesthesiologist
___ Dermatologist
___ Ophthalmologist
___ Otolaryngologist
___ Physiatrist (Rehabilitation Medicine

Career Rating and Preference Inventory (CRAPI)

Code Number ____   Date of Administration _____

Career Rating and Preference Questionnaire

01-02 At this point in your professional development, in what area or specialty of medicine do you plan to work?
_____

Please rate all of the following areas of medicine in terms of your current inclination or disinclination to practice in them. (Mark the number indicating your opinion in the space provided before the titles.) PLEASE USE THE FOLLOWING SCALE:

l=Strongly inclined to avoid   2=Moderately inclined to avoid   3=Slightly inclined to avoid

4=Neither inclined nor disinclined   5=Slightly inclined to select   6=Moderately inclined to select 7=Strongly inclined to select

03 __ Allergy
04 __ Anesthesiology
05 __ Basic Medical Science (e. g., Pharmacology, Physiology)
06 __ Cardiology
07 __ Dermatology
08 __ Family Medicine
09 __ Gastroenterology
10 __ General Practice
11 __ Internal Medicine
12 __ Neurology
13 __ Neurosurgery
14 __ Obstetrics & Gynecology
15 __ Ophthalmology
16 __ Orthopedics

17 __ Otolaryngology
18 __ Pathology
19 __ Pediatrics
20 __ Physical Medicine and Rehabilitation
21 __ Plastic Surgery
22 __ Psychiatry
23 __ Pulmonary diseases
24 __ Public health/preventive medicine
25 __ Radiology
26 __ Thoracic Surgery
27 __ Urology
28 __ Other specialty you would consider: (please specify) _
29 __ General Surgery

How much variety would you prefer to have in a practice with regard to the range of conditions to be dealt with? Rank your 1st, 2nd and 3rd choices:

37 __ Generalized practice
38 __ Moderately specialized
39 __ Highly specialized (sub-specialty)

What is your current inclination or disinclination toward working with each of the following groups? PLEASE USE THE FOLLOWING SCALE:

l=Strongly inclined to avoid   2=Moderately inclined to avoid   3=Slightly inclined to avoid

4=Neither inclined nor disinclined   5=Slightly inclined to select   6=Moderately inclined to select

7=Strongly inclined to select

40 __ Neonate
41 __ Child
42 __ Adolescent
43 __ Adult
44 __ Geriatric Group
45 __ All Ages unselectively

Please rate each of the following career settings in terms of your current inclination or disinclination to work in them. PLEASE USE THE SCALE ABOVE

46 __ Private Practice, solo or partnership
47 __ Private Practice, groups
48 __ Mixed specialty (e. g., small clinic)
49 __ Team practice of one specialty
50 __ Large group (hospital based, e. g., Lovelace Clinic)
51 __ Government Institutions or Agencies
52 __ VA Hospital
53 __ Military Hospital

Physician Career Choice and Satisfaction

54 __ City, State or County Hospital
55 __ City, State or County Health Department
56 __ Public Health Service (non-hospital based)
57 __ Government Sponsored Health Program
58 __ Non-governmental Institutions or Agencies (incl. pharmaceutical co., ins. co., etc.)
59 __ Industry
60 __ Private Hospital (staff physician)
61 __ Independent Medical Foundation (e. g., Kaiser Foundation)
62 __ Research Facility (medical school or any of above)
63 __ Educational Institution (e. g., medical school)

When you have completed your medical education, would you prefer or not prefer to work in a community with the following characteristics? Please rate each characteristic on a seven-point scale where l=strongly inclined to avoid and 7=strongly inclined to prefer.

LOCATION:

27 __ Northwestern United States
28 __ Southeastern United States
29 __ Midwest
30 __ South Central (Texas, Arkansas, Oklahoma)
31 __ Rocky Mountain Stales
32 __ West Coast (Wash., Oregon, Calif., Alaska, Hawaii)
33 __ Foreign (please specify):_____

SIZE OF COMMUNITY

34 __ Over 100,000 population (large metropolitan area)
35 __ Suburban area adjacent to large metropolitan area
36 __ Population between 50,000 and 100,000 (medium city)
37 __ Population between 10,000 and 49,999 (small city)
38 __ Population less than 10,000 (small town or rural)

ECONOMIC STATUS OF COMMUNITY:

39 __ Poverty area or low economic status
40 __ Moderate income area
41 __ Wealthy community

POLITICAL CLIMATE:

42 __ "Liberal"
43 __ Mixed
44 __ "Conservative"

AGE DISTRIBUTION:

45 __ Skewed toward younger age groups
46 __ Skewed toward older age groups

TYPICAL LIFE STYLE OR "PACE"

47 __ Community with a "fast" pace (e. g., New York, L.A., Chi.)
48 __ Community with a "slower" pace of life (e. g., Albuquerque, Tucson)

How often do you use your leisure time in (please indicate highest frequency using the scale below):

Daily | 2-6X/wk | weekly | once/mo |<1/mo | never

    1   2   3   4   5   6

49 __ Meetings of civic, church, political or other task- oriented groups
50 __ Structured recreation groups (such as team sports, bridge clubs, drama clubs)
51 __ Professional groups (having to do with medicine or medical school
52 __ Individual or solitary activity (hobby, sports, music, reading)
53 __ Informal or unstructured outings or entertainment with friends
54 __ Recreation with only family
55 __ Other category {specify)
56 __ Other category {specify)
What is your preferred or most enjoyed leisure time activity, regardless of how often you are able to engage in it?
_____

60 __ Please specify any change in your marital status that has occurred this past school year, where 0=no change; 1=marriage; 2=divorced, separated, widowed.

61 __ Please specify any change in family composition that has occurred this past school year, where 0=no change; 1=addition of a child.

Assuming a position you obtained allowed for a variety of professional activities, what percentage of your time would you like to devote to: *Total responses to 100% of your time*

62 __ Direct Patient Care
63 __ Teaching Medical Personnel
64 __ General Administration
65 __ Program Planning
66 __ Case Consultation
67 __ Professional community service (talks, advisory groups)
68 __ Supervision of Others
69 __ Research
70 __ Other you would include (please specify)

How important do you think each of the following categories of community characteristics will be in your choice of a position or practice setting after completion of your medical training? Please rate each characteristic (category) on a seven-point scale where 1=not at all important-will not consider, and 7=extremely important-crucial to any decision,·

the integers in between represent gradations of importance between these two extremes.

71 __ Geographical location
72 __ Size (population)
73 __ Community Economic Status
74 __ Quality of Public School System
75 __ Age distribution of population
76 __ Ethnic distribution of population
77 __ Political "climate"
78 __ "Pace of Life"
79 __ Distance from metropolitan area
80 __ Distance from a medical school
81 __ Availability of support services (e. g., labs)

Opportunities for:

82 __ Your preferred cultural, recreational or entertainment activities
83 __ Working in your most preferred type of work setting (please see list, question #3)
84 __ Your spouse to obtain employment or pursue a career
85 __ Being in a high demand/low supply specialty for the area
86 __ Proximity to persons prominent in your field of medicine
87 __ Other Characteristics (Please specify):

At this stage in the course of your career, have you, for the most part, stopped considering alternative opportunities in any of the following areas of decision making? That is, do you no longer weigh advantages and disadvantages, or search for new information relevant to a decision? Please place a zero (0) in the space provided alongside each area for which you feel you are still considering alternatives and a one (1) alongside those areas for which you feel you have arrived at a decision.

88 __ Area of Medicine (Specialty)
89 __ Type of practice (e. g., solo, group, institutional)
90 __ Type of work (e. g., clinical, administration, teaching, research)
91 __ Geographic region of practice
92 __ Size of community in which to locate

How important do you think each of the following characteristics of work settings will be in your choice of a position? Please rate each characteristic on a seven-point scale where 1=not at all important-will not consider; and 7=extremely important crucial to any decision: the integers in between represent gradations of importance between these two extremes.

93 __ Income/salary
94 __ Ability to control income (e. g., set fees)
95 __ Job security, benefits
96 __ Type of patients or clients
97 __ Variety of practice activities possible
98 __ Ability to control hours
99 __ Ability to control patient load
100 __ Frequency of need to meet emergencies
101 __ Amount of "red tape" involved in carrying out job activities

102 __ Prestige of organization or group
103 __ Professional abilities of co-workers
104 __ Personal characteristics of co-workers
105 __ Amount of routine task activity

Opportunity for:

106 __ Part-time affiliation with a medical school
107 __ "Getting ahead" professionally
108 __ Directing others in their work
109 __ Molding one's own roles, duties and activities
110 __ Trying out one's own ideas
111 __ Expanding one's own knowledge in an area of medicine
112 __ Working with other physicians on some joint task
113 __ Working with non-physicians in a treatment team
114 __ Other characteristics (Please specify):

Biographical Questionnaire

Code Number _____

Date of Administration _____

BIOGRAPHICAL QUESTIONNAIRE

(1,2) __ Age at entering medical school

Sex

(3-1) __ Male
(3-2) __ Female

Marital Status

(4-1) __ Married
(4-2) __ Single
(4-3) __ Other

(5) __ Number of children

Religion

(6-1) __ Protestant
(6-2) __ Catholic
(6-3) __ Jewish

Physician Career Choice and Satisfaction

(6-4) __ Other
(6-5) __ No Affiliation

How much importance does religion have in your life?

(7-0) __ None
(7-1) __ Very Much
(7-2) __ Some
(7-3) __ A little

Racial Background

(8-1) __ Afro-American, Black
(8-2) __ American-Indian
(8-3) __ Caucasian
(8-4) __ Oriental
(8-5) __ Mex./Sp. American, Chicano
(8-6) __ Puerto-Rican
(8-7) __ Other

State Father's principal occupation. (Please be specific. If businessman or proprietor, please include type and size of business establishment If retired or deceased, indicate last major position.)

_____

Please check what you judge your father's occupational category to be according to the following list:

FATHER:

9-1 __ Higher execs., proprietors of large concerns, and major professionals
9-2 __ Business mgrs., proprietors of medium sized concerns, and lesser professionals
9-3 __ Administrative personnel, small independent business owners, minor professionals
9-4 __ Clerical and sales personnel, technicians, very small business
9-5 __ Skilled manual employees
9-6 __ Machine operators and semi-skilled employees
9-7 __ Unskilled employees
9-8 __ Unemployed

Father's occupational specialty if in a health field

(10-0) __ no medical occupation
(10-1) __ M.D., D.O.
(10-2) __ Dentist
(10-3) __ Nurse
(10-4) __ Other health-med professional

State mother's principal occupation. (Please be specific. If business woman or proprietress, please include size and

type of business establishment. If retired or deceased, indicate last major position)
_____

Please check what you judge your mother's occupational category to be according to the following list:

11-1 __ Higher execs, proprietors of large concerns, and major professionals
11-2 __ Business mgrs., proprietors of medium sized concerns, and lesser professionals
11.3 __ Administrative personnel, small independent business owners, minor professionals
11-4 __ Clerical and sales personnel, technicians, very small business
11-5 __ Skilled manual employees
11-6 __ Machine operators and semi-skilled employees
11-7 __ Unskilled employees
11-8 __ Housewife or unemployed

Mother's occupational specialty if in a health field

(12-0) __ no medical occupation
(12-1) __ M.D., D.O.
(12-2) __ Dentist
(12-3) __ Nurse
(12-4) __ Other health-med professional

Parents' education (check only highest level for each parent):

FATHER: MOTHER:

(13-1) __ (14-1) __ Graduate or professional training beyond college
(13-2) __ (14-2) __ Graduated from college only
(13-3) __ (14-3) __ Attended college but did not graduate or attended a vocational or trade school beyond high school
(13-4) __ (14-4) __ Graduated from high school only
(13-5) __ (14-5) __ Attended high school but did not finish (10, 11, some 12th gr)
(13--6) __ (14-6) __ Attended jr. high school (7, 8, or 9th gr)
(13-7) __ (14-7) __ Less than 7 years
(13-8) __ (14-8) __ No formal education

Estimate of parents' average annual income before taxes: [pre-retirement or average income when working)

(15-1) __ Less than $5,000
(15-2) __ $5,000 to $9,999
(15-3) __ $10,000 to $14,999
(15-4) __ $15,000 to $24,999
(15-5) __ $25,000 to $49,999
(15-6) __ $50,000 to $99,999
(15-7) __ $100,000 or more

Please check (\/) the appropriate spaces (on the following page) indicating community size and geographic region for

Physician Career Choice and Satisfaction

the places you lived from ages 0-7; 8-13; and 14-18. Refer to the size and geographic region categories shown below. If you lived in more than one place during any age period, check the one where you lived the longest.

*Community Size:

1. Large metropolitan area (500,000 or more) including suburbs of 100,000 or more
2. Moderately sized community (25,000- 99,999)
3. Small town (24,999 or less)

**Geographic Region:

1. MIDWEST (Mich., Minn., Wis., Iowa, 111., Ind., ND, SD, Neb., Kan)
2. NORTHEAST (Me., NH, Vt., Mass., RI, Conn., NY, Pa., Ohio, Md., NJ, Del., DC)
3. WEST COAST (Cal., Ore., Wash., Alaska, Hawaii) J
4. ROCKY MOUNTAIN (NM, Ariz., Colo., Utah, Nev., Wyo., Mont., Idaho)
5. SOUTH-SOUTHEAST (Va., W.Va., Tenn., Ky., Ark., NC, SC, Ga., Fla., Ala., Miss., La., Tex., Okla., Mo.)
6. FOREIGN COUNTRY

Age 0-7

Comm. Size 16-1 __ 16-2 __ 16-3 __
Geog. Region** 17-1 __ 17-2 __ 17-3 __ 17-4 __ 17-5 __ 17-6 __

Age 8-13

Comm. Size. 18-1 __ 18-2 __ 18-3 __
Geog. Region** 19-1 __ 19-2 __ 19-3 __ 19-4 __ 19-5 __ 19-6 __

Age 14-18

Comm. Size. 20-1 __ 20-2 __ 20-3 __
Geog. Region** 21-1 __ 21-2 __ 21-3 __ 21-4 __ 21-5 __ 21-6 __
Number of male children in your family (include yourself): (22) _

Number of female children in your family (include yourself): (23) _

Your position among your siblings:

24-7 __ Only child
24-2 __ Oldest of 2
24-3 __ Youngest of 2
24-4 __ Oldest of 3
24-5 __ Middle of 3
24-6 __ Youngest of 3
24-7 __ O1dest of 4 or more
24-8 __ Middle of 4 or more

24-9 __ Youngest of 4 or more

Undergraduate colleges attended (for longer than summer session.) List first the one you graduated from most recently or most recently attended:

NAME OF SCHOOL	STATE:	Public	Private
_____ 25	_____ 26-1	_____ 26-2	_____
_____ 27	_____ 28-1	_____ 28-2	_____
_____ 29	_____ 30-1	_____ 30-2	_____

Undergraduate major and minor areas:

Major

31,32-01 __ Biological Sciences
02 __ Physical Science
03 __ Social Sciences
04 __ Humanities
05 __ Fine Arts/ Architecture
06 __ Education
07 __ Engineering
08 __ Business
09 __ Economics
10 __ Health Professions
11 __ Home Economics
12 __ Other
13 __ No major (e. g. University College)
35-7 __ Pre-med; Pre-law; Pre-dentistry; etc.

Minor

33,34-01 __
02 __
03 __
04 __
05 __
06 __
07 __
08 __
09 __
10 __
11 __
12 __
13 __

Using the list of subjects above, please indicate which two subjects you enjoyed most and which two subjects you enjoyed least, as an undergraduate, by writing the appropriate numbers in the spaces below (e.g., 01 =Biological Sciences, 02=Physical Sciences, etc.)

Enjoyed most

36,37 __ 38,39 __

Enjoyed least

40,4] __ 42,43 __

Graduate Schools attended, if any (if more than one, list most recent FIRST):

NAME OF SCHOOL   STATE: Public   Private

Physician Career Choice and Satisfaction

_____ 44 _____ 45-1 _____ 45-2 _____
_____ 46 _____ 47-1 _____ 47-2 _____
_____ 48 _____ 49-1 _____ 49-2 _____

Graduate major and minor areas:

Major   Minor

50,51-01 __ Biological Sciences   52,53-01 __
02 __ Physical Science   02 __
03 __ Social Sciences   03 __
04 __ Humanities   04 __
05 __ Fine Arts/ Architecture   05 __
06 __ Education   06 __
07 __ Engineering   07 __
08 __ Business   08 __
09 __ Economics   09 __
10 __ Health Professions   10 __
11 __ Home Economics   11 __
12 __ Other   12 __
13 __ No major (e. g. University College)   13 __

Current educational status:

54-07 __ Less than BA or BS
02 __ Bachelor's Degree
03 __ Bachelor's+ grad. hrs.
04 __ MA or MS degree
05 __ MA or MS+ additional hrs.
06 __ All but thesis for PhD
07 __ PhD-MD-Grad. Degree: EdD, DDS, etc.

Type of doctoral degree if any:

55-0 __ no doctoral
55-1 __ PhD
55-2 __ MD
55-3 __ OD
55-4 __ DDS
55-5 __ EdD

Please indicate up to 4 areas in which you have had occupational or organizational experience prior to entry into medical school:

56-__   57-__   58-__   59-__

__(0) no experience
__(1) Experience in medical care setting, e. g., working in a hospital, ambulance attendant, work in clinical laboratory (but not a research lab), etc.
__(2) Experience in "helping" activities, e. g., counselor, playground director, social casework, work with under-

privileged children or adults, work with juvenile corrections, Peace Corps, VISTA, etc.
___(3) Research or Technical experience, e. g., lab technician, biologist, engineer, technical aide, research assistant, etc.
___(4) Teaching experience, e. g., instructor, .tutor, graduate assistant, etc.
___(5) Experience in dealing with the public, e. g., salesman, public affairs officer, etc.
___(6) Unskilled labor, e. g., construction work, life guard, receptionist, work in summer resorts, checker in grocery store, etc.
___ (7) Other (specify): ----------------------------

60 ___ How many medical schools did you apply to?

61 ___ Where did University of New Mexico rank in your preference of schools you applied to?

Have you ever made application to a medical school before this year?

62-0 ___ No, have not applied before this year
62-1 ___ Yes, have made application once before
62-2 ___ Yes, have made application in two or more previous years

Please indicate by a 1, 2, or 3 the importance to you of the following factors in having selected this particular medical school (where 1 = no importance, 2 = some importance, and 3 = much importance):

___ 01 Liked idea of attending a medical school that was newly established.
___ 02 Liked idea of attending a medical school that was well established.
___ 03 Liked the sound of the program (curriculum) to be offered at this school.
___ 04 Wanted to live in this area.
___ 05 Needed to live in this area (for financial or other reasons).
___ 06 Liked clinical emphasis in the program.
___ 07 Liked research emphasis in the program.
___ 08 Liked the size of the school.
___ 09 Liked the attitudes of students and faculty.
___ 10 Faculty has a good reputation.
___ 11 Was impressed by the facilities available.
___ 12 Was influenced by friend(s) to attend this school.
___ 13 Was influenced by parents or spouse to attend this school.
___ 14 Was influenced by physician friend(s) to attend this medical school.
___ 15 Was influenced by faculty or staff member to attend this medical school.
___ 16 Only medical school at which accepted.
___ 17 Other (specify):----------------------------

Medical School Graduates Survey

CODE NUMBER: _____

DATE: _____

Physician Career Choice and Satisfaction

MEDICAL SCHOOL GRADUATES SURVEY

The following questions are designed to gather information related to experience you have had since graduation. Please answer questions that are directed toward programs you are in or have completed. Skip over items that are not applicable to your situation.

1. Present age ____

2. Marital Status: ___Married ___Single ___Other (specify)

3. Spouse's Occupation _____

4. Number of Children ____

5. Religion;   ___ Protestant   ___ Jewish

   ___ Catholic   ___ Other

6. How much importance does religion have in your life: ___Very much   ___A little

   ___Some   ___None

7. Internship entry date (month, year) _____

8. Name of Institution _____

9. Type of Internship program (please check one):

   Straight Medicine ___   Rotating ___
   Straight Obstetrics-Gyn ___
   Straight Pathology ___
   Straight Pediatrics ___
   Straight Surgery ___
   Please specify services in the order of rotation: _____
   Other (please specify) _____

10. Which rank was this institution among your application choices?

    1st ___ 2nd ___ 3rd ___ 4th or below ___

11. To how many places did you apply (or rank in the matching program)? ____

12. Residency entry date (month, year) (specify if resiternship) _____

13. Name of Institution _____

14. Specialty Training in _____

15. Length of program _____

16. Which rank was this institution among your application choices?

1st ___ 2nd ___ 3rd ___ 4th or below ___

17. To how many places did you apply?____

18. Did any person(s) assist in getting you an internship? ___Yes ___ No ___Don't Know

    Residency placement? ___ Yes ___ No ___ Don't Know

19. Please estimate the *amount of time* during internship and residency spent in the following types of institutions (indicate by a check if any were also University affiliated institutions/ programs):

	Internship		Residency	
	Inpatient	Outpatient (clinics)	Inpatient	Outpatient (clinics)
Private Hospital				
City/County Hospital				
State Hospital				
VA System				
Public Health Service				
Military Facility				
University Facility				
Other (specify)				

20. What is your status with regard to the military? (Check appropriate category)

    ___ Draft or service exempt (e. g., female, 4F)
    ___ No plans or commitment as yet
    ___ Requirement completed
    ___ Currently under military assignment
    ___ Commitment for future has been made (please explain the arrangement, e. g., Berry plan):
    _____

21. Do you have a government service obligation period due to a previous or present stipend?

    ___ No ___ Yes

    If so, what is your payback requirement? _____

Physician Career Choice and Satisfaction

22. If you have completed or are currently in a military or government service program, please specify:

Date of service entry _____
Length of program _____
Title and Type of program (please explain): _____
Training plan if any (e. g., residency, internship) _____
Name of Service Institution(s) _____
Payback requirement, if any _____

23. Were you drafted? __ Yes __No   If so, when? _____

24. What do you see as the advantages offered by the military program you have selected?

_____

_____

25. If your time since UNM graduation is not classifiable as internship, residency or military service, what have you been up to?

_____

_____

26. During your post graduate training, how frequently did your supervisors observe you doing medical tasks:

	During Internship	During Residency
Daily		
More than once/wk.		
Once/wk.		
Two-four times/wk.		
Once/month		
Bimonthly		
Less than every 2 months		

27. How frequently did your supervisors demonstrate methods or techniques to you?

	During Internship	During Residency
Daily		
More than once/wk.		
Once/wk.		
Two-four times/wk.		
Once/month		

Bimonthly		
Less than every 2 months		

28. How frequently did your supervisors assist you in working out problems of patient care?

	During Internship	During Residency
Daily		
More than once/wk.		
Once/wk.		
Two-four times/wk.		
Once/month		
Bimonthly		
Less than every 2 months		

29. To what extent have your supervisors discussed with you your professional strengths and weaknesses?

	During Internship	During Residency
Not at all		
Slightly		
A fair amount		
A great deal		

30. How formalized were the evaluations you received?

	During Internship	During Residency
Regularly scheduled and designed to cover specific areas		
Regularly scheduled but without a specific plan		
Scheduled when requested but with no formal plan		
Haphazard, no formal evaluations		

31. How satisfied have you been with the amount of evaluation you received?

	During Internship	During Residency

Very satisfied		
Moderately well satisfied		
Satisfied		
Mildly dissatisfied		
Very dissatisfied		

32. How consistent has the feedback been regarding your performance?

	During Internship	During Residency
Very consistent		
Mostly consistent		
Very inconsistent		

33. How many different individuals have served as coaches or critics to you, personally, during Internship? (enter number):___ During Residency? ___

34. The following group s might, at one time or another, judge the quality of professional performance. Whose judgments, in your opinion, should count most when your overall professional performance is assessed? (Please rank 1st, 2nd and 3rd beside the appropriate group -- add groups if the list does not satisfy you.)

Rank	Group
	Interns/residents
	Attending physicians
	Patients and/or families
	Your own family
	Your former medical school faculty
	Nurses
	The community
	Others in the health care field (Specify)_____

35. At what stage in the course of your career did you, for the most part, stop considering alternative opportunities in the following areas of decision-making? That is, when did you no longer weigh advantages and disadvantages or search for new information relevant to a decision? Please check the appropriate box below each decision area:

	Decision Area				
	Specialty (area of	Type of Practice	Type of work (e. g., clinical,	Geographic region of	Size of community to

Stage	medicine)	(solo, group, etc.)	admin., research, etc)	practice	locate in
Prior to medical school					
By end of 2nd year med. school					
By end of medical school					
By end of internship					
By end of military obligation (if prior to residency)					
By end of 1st year of residency					
By middle of residency					
By end of residency					
By end of military obligation					
Still working on this decision					

36. When applying for your internship and residency, to what extent did you pay attention to the following factors?

Factor	Internship				Residency			
	None	Slight	A lot	Great deal	None	Slight	A lot	Great deal
Salary								
Call schedule								
Characteristics of geographic location								
Staff-patient ratio of the institution								
Reputation of institution								
Breadth of programs								
Specific program emphasis								
Affiliation with medical school								
Opportunity to work under an established medical figure								
Availability of research facilities								
Size of institution								
Patient population characteristics								

Following advice or footsteps of a respected mentor							
Suitability of geographical area for future practice							
Opportunity to work with people already known							
Amount of individual freedom given to trainees							
Degree of structure of training program							
Opportunity to make "contacts" for the future							
Familiarity with the geographic region							
Opportunity for staying where I was							
Opportunities available for my spouse's pursuits							
Opportunity to go someplace else							
Amount of patient responsibility afforded the house staff							
General feeling of "rightness" about the place							
Reputation of potential colleagues							
Other (Please specify: _____)							

37. Not all possibilities for choice are open to everyone in choosing internships and residencies. How much did the factors listed below limit your internship/residency placement? (check the degree for each constraint)

Factor	Internship				Residency			
	None	Slight	A lot	Great deal	None	Slight	A lot	Great deal
EXTERNAL CONSTRAINTS: Family needs for a particular location (health, special education, etc)								
Pressing financial considerations								
Limiting academic record								
Uninspiring letters of recommendation								

Over supply of applicants for preferred specialty or institution								
Spouse's preferences								
Funding cutbacks to institutions (decrease in positions available)								
Pre-established path commitment (e. g., prior military enrollment/training)								
Limited information at choice points (Didn't know all that was available)								
Other (Please specify)								
FIXED PERSONAL DESIRES Climate or geography preference								
Distance (near/far) from family/friends								
Desire for "change of scene"								
Desire not to relocate								
Life style requirements (recreational needs, church association, etc.)								
Other (Please specify)								

38. What are your plans for the immediate future (1-2 years)?

_____

_____

_____

_____

39. What (if anything) stands out in your mind as having influenced you (positively or negatively) in the direction of your current plans?

Physician Career Choice and Satisfaction

_____
_____
_____
_____

40. What task(s) in medicine have you found to be the most enjoyable to you so far?
_____

_____
_____
_____
_____

41. In light of your present situation, in what ways would you have liked your undergraduate medical school education to have been different?
_____
_____
_____

Physician Work Setting Instrument (PWSI)

Respondent No. _____

Physician Work Setting Instrument

This questionnaire is designed to gather information about the variety of work settings within which physicians practice. Emphasis is placed upon your present medical setting. To get some perspective on the direction of your medical career, there are a few questions about the settings in which you *previously* practiced medicine

GENERAL INFORMATION

1. Sex ___ Male ___ Female

2. Marital Status ___ Married ___ Unmarried

3. Religion ___ Protestant ___ Jewish ___ Catholic ___ Other

4. Size of community where you spent the majority of your pre-college years:

(a) ___ under 10,000 population   (b) ___ 10,000-49,000   (c) ___ 50,000-100,000,

(d) __ 100,000 -999,000   (e) ___ over 1,000,000

5. Type of internship; STRAIGHT: __ Medicine __ Surgery .___Ob-Gyn __ Pathology ___ Pediatrics
        ROTATING: _____OTHER: (Specify) _____

6. Specialty training: __ Yes __ No

7. If yes, in which medical specialty (or specialties)? _____

PREVIOUS MEDICAL WORK SETTINGS

Please include all work settings after graduation from medical school, including internship, residency and military service as a physician. Please refer to the "Types of Settings" and "Reasons for changing settings" by the numbers indicated on the list below. Give as many reasons for change as are relevant.

	Type of Setting	Years in Setting	Reasons for Change		Type of Setting	Years in Setting	Reasons for Change
Internship				Fifth			
Residency				Sixth			
Required military or alternates				Seventh			
Fourth				Eighth			

Types of Settings

1. Solo practice
2. Partnership
3. Solo with arrangement with other physicians
4. Small group practice (6 or less); same specialty
5. Small group practice (mixed specialties)
6. Large group practice (7 or more)
7. Large group with hospital-based facility
8. Medical School
9. Hospital: Specify (a) non-government, (b) city/county, (c) state, (d) military, (e) VA
10. Public Health Service
11. Other _____

Reasons for changing past work settings

1. General dissatisfaction with professional position or setting
2. Opportunity for expanded medical role (e. g., more diverse tasks) in the new setting
3. Opportunity for concentrating on one or a few areas of maximal interest
4. Opportunity for more enjoyable activities; different responsibilities, etc.
5. Opportunity to relocate-in a more desirable professional area [more services, better hospitals)
6. Opportunity to treat patients with different characteristics
7. Availability of a better professional situation (increased salary, higher level position, etc.)
8. General family life style considerations
9. "System Frustration" associated with the previous setting (red tape, regulations, etc.)
10. Unresolvable differences with colleagues or superiors in previous setting
11. Opportunity to-follow a slower pace in the new setting
12. Obligation was completed, e. g., internship, residency, military (Please give additional reasons if they apply)

Physician Career Choice and Satisfaction

13. Desire for further training
14. Other (Specify) _____

CHANGE IN SPECIALTY

Have you ever changed your specialty area? __ Yes __ No
IF YES: What was your original specialty? _____
At what point in your career did the change in specialty occur?
(a) After __ years of residency   (b) After __ years of practice

PRESENT WORK-SETTING

1. Primary setting (Use numbered list below) ___ If you work in more than one type of' setting on a regular basis, please indicate and/or briefly describe your circumstances:
_____
_____

Types of Settings

1. Solo practice
2. Partnership
3. Solo with arrangement with other physicians
4. Small group practice or less); same specialty
5. Small group practice (mixed specialties)
6. Large group practice (7 or more)
7. Large group with hospital-based facility
8. Medical School
9. Hospital: Specify (a) non-government, (b) city/county, (c) state, (d) military, (e) VA
10. Public Health Service
11. Other _____

2. Length of time in setting (if more than one, length of time in major setting) _____ years.

3. Which of the following best describes your patient drawing area? (Please circle)

a) designated neighborhood   b) town, city or borough of metropolitan area

c) suburban area   d) town and surrounding rural area   e) county   f) state

g) Other (specify) _____

4. Present income from medicine only: a) less than 20,000/yr. b) 20,000--29,000 c) 30,000-39,000

d) 40,000-49,000 e) 50,000/more

Patient Characteristics

5. Predominant age(s): __ Neonate __ Adolescent __ Geriatric __ Child __ Adult __ All
6. Sex: (Primarily) __ Males __ Females __ Both
7. Income level: (Primarily) __ Low Income __ Middle Income __ High Income __ Mixture
8. Ethnic background (Primarily) __ Black __ Caucasian __ Mexican/Spanish American __ Puerto Rican __ American Indian __ Mixture of racial backgrounds _____ Other

9. Percent (approximate) of your total patients who are referred to you by other physicians ___ %
10. Percent (approximate) of your total patients whom you refer to other physicians ___ %
11. Average number of patients seen per week ___.

Activities and Characteristics

The major information we are seeking concerns (a) activities and characteristics associated with physician work settings and (b) how these activities and characteristics contribute to the satisfaction and dissatisfaction of physicians. The following two sections, *Professional Activities* and *Setting Characteristics* are designed to provide both kinds of information by a single score for each item.

Professional Activities

For each activity listed, select the *frequency category* (i. e., daily, weekly, etc) that indicates how often you now perform the activity. Then, in the selected frequency box, indicate how often you *would like* to perform the activity by a plus (+) if you would like to do it *more often*; a minus (-) if you would like to do it *less often*; an equal sign (=) if you would like to do it with the *same* frequency; and an (x) if it is irrelevant (i. e., you don't care how often you do it).

Example A shows that "performing lab tests" is done on a weekly basis and that the physician would like to do it *less frequently*. Example B shows that "attending medical society meetings" is done on a yearly basis and that the physician would like to continue doing it with the *same frequency*. Using this method of notation, please complete all of the activity items listed.

ACTIVITIES	Daily	Weekly	Monthly	Yearly	Never
A. Performing lab tests		(-)			
B. Attending medical society meetings				(=)	
1. Case consultation with other professional personnel					
2. Supervision and/or teaching medical students or medical personnel (e. g., paramedics)					
3. Providing some form of patient care outside of the major practice setting (e. g., community clinics, hospitals)					
4. Performing diagnostic procedures, including lab tests, upper G.I. Series, biopsies, cytologies, autopsies, etc.)					
5. Performing therapeutic procedures, including surgery, psychotherapy, radiologic treatment, etc.					
6. Presenting cases to some audience					
7. Reviewing patient charts, including analysis of test results.					
8. Explaining diagnoses and treatment plans to patients and their families.					
9. Organizational administration (e. g., committee work, policy development)					

Physician Career Choice and Satisfaction

10. Testifying in court in medical-legal proceedings						
11. Reading journals and medical books						
12. Assisting other physicians in performing procedures						
13. Referring patients to other practitioners or institutions						
14. Medical record keeping						
15. Other activity not included (Please describe) _____						

Setting Characteristics

For each item listed, select the category indicating the degree to which it is characteristic of your present work situation (i. e., very *un*characteristic through very characteristic). Then, in the selected box, indicate whether you *would like* this factor to be *more* characteristic (+); *less* characteristic (-); the *same* (=); or whether it is *irrelevant* (x), i. e., it doesn't matter.

Example A shows that "Determining breadth of activities" is *slightly characteristic* and that the physician would like it to be *more* characteristic (+). Example B shows that "filling out insurance forms" is *very* characteristic, and that the physician would like it to be *less* characteristic (-). Using this method of notation, please complete all of the items listed.

Items	Uncharacteristic			Characteristic		
	Very	Moderate	Slight	Slight	Moderate	Very
A. Determining breadth of activities				(+)		
B. Filling out insurance forms						(-)
1. Responsibility for defining one's role, duties and activities						
2. Personal control of amount of time devoted to patient care						
3. Supervision of subordinates						
4. Trying out new ideas						
5. Expanding one's own knowledge in an area of medicine						
6. Serious financial constraints limiting provision of patient care						
7. Dealing with patient's emotional difficulties						
8. Working with other physicians on some joint task						
9. Access to new developments in a field of interest or specialization						

10. Dealing with new or unusual patient problems						
11. Sharing patient responsibility with other physicians						
12. Paperwork						
13. Working with paraprofessionals or physician extenders						
14. Emphasis on diagnosing and developing treatment plans						
15. Maintaining a fairly consistent and predictable patient scheduling system						
16. Dealing with emergency medical problems						
17. Personal control of amount of earnings						
18. Access to hospital facilities						
19. Opportunity for affiliation with a medical school						
20. Focus on special interest area within a specialty						
21. Opportunity for professional advancement						
22. Teaching medical students, interns or residents						
23. Intellectual stimulation through interaction with colleagues						
24. Performing habitual or non-varying medical activities						
25. Working alone (little assistance from other medical personnel)						
26. Delegation of certain medical tasks to subordinates						
27. Devoting time to particular patient problems or kinds of patients						
28. Satisfactory coverage for patients during times of absence						
29. Personally handling financial aspects of medical practice						
30. Dealing with ethical or moral issues in the practice of medicine						
31. Opportunity to follow and evaluate patient progress						
32. Sharing doubts, frustrations or problems with colleagues						
33. Advising or counseling patients and/or their families						
34. Opportunity for appreciation and prestige from the lay public						
35. Accessibility of consultation services						

Physician Career Choice and Satisfaction

36. Isolation from other physicians						
37. Direct patient contact						
38. Opportunity for prestige and recognition from colleagues						
39. Time "wasted" due to travel between professional locations						
40. Working with or under a community board or citizens group						
41. Taking less vacation and/or free time than one is entitled to take						
42. Maintaining my preferred "pace of life"						
43. Determining amount of free time and/or vacation time						
44. Sufficient time for family and/or outside activities						
45. Cultural or recreational activities in my geographical area						
46. Availability of desirable public school system						
47. Opportunities for spouse to be employed or pursue preferred activities						
48. Active participation in non-medical community affairs						

Evaluation of Present Work Situation

Examining distinct activities and characteristics of a work setting may not accurately reflect a physician's judgment of his total situation. That is, "the whole may be different than the sum of its parts." In light of this, please circle the statements below which best describe your assessment of your work situation.

(1.) I am very satisfied with both my specialty and my work setting.
(2) I would probably be more satisfied in a different specialty area but my work setting is very satisfactory (SEE-"EXPLANATIONS" LIST BELOW)
(3) I am satisfied with my specialty, but my work setting is unsatisfactory. (SEE "EXPLANATIONS" LIST BELOW)
(4) I am dissatisfied with both my specialty and work setting. (SEE "EXPLANATIONS" LIST'BELOW)

Explanations

Please select the appropriate explanation(s) from the list below:

(1) I *am* contemplating a change in setting and/or specialty in the near future.
(2) I am not contemplating a change in specialty or work setting in the near future because:
    (a) It is impractical at this time (financial considerations, family factors, etc.)
    (b) My present situation allows me to devote a lot of time to favorite non-professional activities.
    (c) I am not dissatisfied enough to make any major change(s) in the near future.
    (d) Other _____

Gerald Otis and Naomi Quenk

The Relationship of Settings to Specialties

Please check the appropriate item:

____I regard my work setting-and my specialty as two distinct aspects of my career. That is, a decision in one area may be made fairly independently of a decision in the other area.

____I regard my work setting and my specialty as interdependent. I don't find it possible or practical to separate specialty from work setting decisions.

ABOUT THE AUTHORS

Gerald D. Otis, PhD, was born in Northfield, Minnesota. He graduated from Northfield High School, attended St. Olaf College for two years, and graduated from the University of Minnesota. He earned his PhD. in Psychology from the University of Arizona in 1966. After completing a clinical internship at the Veterans Administration Hospital in Palo Alto, California he joined the University of New Mexico School of Medicine where he did clinical work, teaching and research. He headed the Longitudinal Study research team in the study of the career decision making process of medical students and physicians and was subsequently the Director of the American Medical Student Association Foundation Center for Physician Career Development, headquartered in Albuquerque.

For 10 years after Dr. Otis left the University, he combined a private practice with the design and construction of sculptural furniture and computer programming. During his years as a psychologist he published results of research on incidental learning, interaction of stress and personality, family psychotherapy, physician career choice, psychological type and the Myers-Briggs Type Indicator, post-traumatic stress disorder, and trends in violent death. He has received two awards from the Association for Psychological Type and several awards for his efforts at fine woodworking.

Following 16 years working for the Veterans Administration in Medford, Oregon, where he specialized in the treatment of post-traumatic stress disorder, Dr. Otis retired from clinical practice and now lives in Las Cruces, New Mexico with his wife Connie. Since retirement, he has authored four books: *Joseph Lee Heywood: His Life and Tragic Death* (biography), *Paroxysm: Love, Murder and Justice in Post Civil War Washington, DC.* (historical novel), *Presumed Crazy: A Fisherman Gets Entangled in the Mental Health Gulag* (exposé) and the present *Physician Career Choice and Satisfaction*.

Naomi L. Quenk, PhD, is a psychologist, author, editor, and independent consultant living in southern Maine. She was an esteemed collaborator on the Longitudinal Study and the Center for Physician Career Development. She has authored or co-authored numerous articles and books on psychological type including, *Types of family practice teachers and residents, Characteristics of physician work settings in relation to Myers-Briggs Preferences; Beside Ourselves: Our Hidden Personality in Everyday Life. Interpretive Guide for the MBTI Expanded Analysis Report, Dream Thinking: The logic, magic, and meaning of dreams, MBTI Step II Expanded Interpretive Report; Manual: A Guide to the development and use of the Myers-Briggs Type Indicator; Essentials of Myers-Briggs Type Indicator Assessment; In the grip: Understanding type, stress, and the inferior function; MBTI Step II Manual: Exploring the next level of type with the Myers-Briggs Type Indicator Form Q; Myers-Briggs Type Indicator Step II Interpretive Report; Was that really me? How everyday stress brings out our hidden personality; Understanding your MBTI Step II Results: A step-by-step guide to your unique expression of type, MBTI® Step III™ Manual: Exploring personality development using the Myers-Briggs Type Indicator® instrument.*, and *MBTI Manual for the Global Step I™* and *Step II™ Assessments*. She won an award for her work on developing the MBTI Step III instrument

www.ingramcontent.com/pod-product-compliance
Lightning Source LLC
Chambersburg PA
CBHW050747100426
42744CB00012BA/1926